Understanding Research for Nursing Students

Sara Miller McCune founded SAGE Publishing in 1965 to support the dissemination of usable knowledge and educate a global community. SAGE publishes more than 1000 journals and over 800 new books each year, spanning a wide range of subject areas. Our growing selection of library products includes archives, data, case studies and video. SAGE remains majority owned by our founder and after her lifetime will become owned by a charitable trust that secures the company's continued independence.

Los Angeles | London | New Delhi | Singapore | Washington DC | Melbourne

Understanding Research for Nursing Students

5E

Peter Ellis

Learning Matters
A SAGE Publishing Company
1 Oliver's Yard
55 City Road
London EC1Y 1SP

SAGE Publications Inc.
2455 Teller Road
Thousand Oaks, California 91320

SAGE Publications India Pvt Ltd
B 1/I 1 Mohan Cooperative Industrial Area
Mathura Road
New Delhi 110 044

SAGE Publications Asia-Pacific Pte Ltd
3 Church Street
#10-04 Samsung Hub
Singapore 049483

Editor: Laura Walmsley
Development editor: Richenda Milton-Daws
Senior project editor: Chris Marke
Project management: River Editorial
Marketing manager: Ruslana Khatagova
Cover design: Sheila Tong
Typeset by: C&M Digitals (P) Ltd, Chennai, India
Printed in the UK

Library of Congress Control Number: 2022930441

British Library Cataloguing in Publication Data

A catalogue record for this book is available from the British Library

ISBN 978-1-5297-7969-1
ISBN 978-1-5297-7968-4 (pbk)

At SAGE we take sustainability seriously. Most of our products are printed in the UK using responsibly sourced papers and boards. When we print overseas we ensure sustainable papers are used as measured by the PREPS grading system. We undertake an annual audit to monitor our sustainability.

Contents

TRANSFORMING NURSING PRACTICE

Transforming Nursing Practice is a series tailor made for pre-registration student nurses. Each book addresses a core topic and is:

 Clearly written and easy to read

 Mapped to the NMC Standards of proficiency for registered nurses

 Full of case studies and activities

 Focused on applying everyday nursing theory to practice

An invaluable series of books that explicitly relates to the NMC standards. Each book covers a different topic that students need to explore in order to develop into a qualified nurse... I would recommend this series to all Pre-Registered nursing students whatever their field or year of study.

LINDA ROBSON,
Senior Lecturer at Edge Hill University

Many titles in the series are on our recommended reading list and for good reason - the content is up to date and easy to read. These are the books that actually get used beyond training and into your nursing career.

EMMA LYDON,
Adult Student Nursing

ABOUT THE SERIES EDITORS

DR MOOI STANDING is an Independent Academic Nursing Consultant (UK and international) responsible for the core knowledge, personal and professional learning skills titles. She has invaluable experience as an NMC Quality Assurance Reviewer of educational programmes, and as a Professional Regulator Panellist on the NMC Practice Committee. Mooi is also a Board member of Special Olympics Malaysia.

DR SANDRA WALKER is a Clinical Academic in Mental Health working between North Bristol Trust and Southern Health Trust. She is series editor for the mental health nursing titles. She is a Qualified Mental Health Nurse with a wide range of clinical experience spanning 30 years and spent several years working as a mental health lecturer at Southampton University.

BESTSELLING TEXTBOOKS

You can find a full list of textbooks in the *Transforming Nursing Practice* series at
uk.sagepub.com/TNP-series

About the author

Peter Ellis is an independent nursing and health and social care writer and consultant, and CEO of Intelligent Care Software. Peter was most recently a registered manager and nursing director in the hospice and social care settings. Prior to this, he was a senior lecturer and programme director at Canterbury Christ Church University where he taught understanding research, among other topics, to undergraduate and postgraduate nursing students. Peter is also an honorary senior research fellow of Canterbury Christ Church University and has a special interest, including ongoing research, in palliative and end-of-life care.

Foreword

The Transforming Nursing Practice series includes several titles that focus on personal and professional learning skills which are mapped against the Standards of Proficiency for Registered Nurses (NMC 2018a), and *Understanding Research for Nursing Students* is a key text in this respect.

On a personal level, it offers students opportunities to gain confidence by getting to grips with important aspects of the research process in nursing. On a professional level, it succinctly demonstrates how a wide range of research methods are used to generate knowledge that can be applied to enhance the quality of care that service users receive. It promotes an awareness of uncertainty, of what we do not know and what we need to find out in order to provide the best care possible. In this way, the book encourages students to adopt a healthy, questioning, evidence-based approach in delivering safe and effective person-centred care. This also goes hand in hand with lifelong learning and their continuing personal and professional development as nurses.

The book gives lots of practical examples and illustrations to help readers relate to the topic, and there are numerous learning activities to engage with, test out ideas and deepen understanding. Helpful additional learning resources are recommended at the end of each chapter for readers to access and clarify their understanding of research concepts further, if they so wish. This complements the author's informative, lucid, interactive and reader friendly style which both nursing students and their lecturers have highly commended.

In the fifth edition of this very popular book, Peter Ellis has updated references, learning activities and contents to reflect recent developments and challenges in healthcare provision, such as COVID-19. This emphasises the importance of scientific research in the epidemiology of disease, developing vaccines through clinical trials, informing public health interventions, providing Personal Protective Equipment, evaluating patients' responses to treatment, and managing a tension between 'putting patients first' and 'protecting the NHS'. It highlights how the knowledge base informing nursing is continually developing and that nurses must be research-minded and keep up to date in order to enhance their practice.

After reading this book, students should have a good grasp of research that will help them both in their academic work and in contributing to high-quality, evidence-based and person-centred nursing care.

Dr Mooi Standing
Series Editor

Introduction

The purpose of this book is to introduce you, the nursing student, to the key concepts involved in nursing and healthcare research. The aim of introducing research is two-fold: the first is to enable you to better understand the research you read to inform your practice and to make some judgements about its quality. The second is to prepare you to undertake research either as part of your role at work or as part of a course of study. Many nurses believe that understanding research, let alone undertaking research, is beyond them. This book sets out to explode this myth by demonstrating that the processes involved in the design and undertaking of research are easily understood.

Understanding Research for Nursing Students does not contain all that any budding researcher will need in order to design and carry out their own research, but it does provide a reasonable overview and suggests other sources of information that may help in the study design process. Clearly, books such as this present an idealistic view of research which, like clinical nursing, is subject to practical considerations and the realities of funding, experience and ability, and so rarely proceeds in a textbook manner.

Chapter 1 introduces what research in health and social care is about, and the sorts of questions that nursing research can be used to answer. It also introduces some of the philosophical assumptions that underpin research, including those that inform the quantitative and qualitative paradigms. The reader is introduced to the processes that a researcher might go through in order to generate a research question. In addition, Chapter 1 introduces the key ethical principles and ideas that inform all phases of the research process. It is important for any researcher to understand and take heed of these issues in the design of a research study in order to design a study that is both realistic and ethical.

Chapters 2 and 3 introduce qualitative research methodologies and methods. Chapter 2 concentrates on identifying the qualitative research methodologies, the questions they set out to answer, the sampling methods they use and the key methods (data collection tools) they employ. Chapter 3 continues the qualitative theme, exploring in more detail the key methods used in qualitative data collection. It goes on to explore some of the issues in data management and analysis of qualitative data.

Chapters 4 and 5 explore the quantitative research methodologies and some research methods. Chapter 4 mirrors Chapter 2 in introducing the quantitative research methodologies, the research questions they set out to answer, the ways in which samples for study are chosen and the key data collection methods they use. Chapter 4 concludes by introducing some of the key methods in data presentation and analysis used in the quantitative research methodologies. Chapter 5 continues to explore the quantitative theme, presenting some of the main methods nurses use when employing the quantitative methods in their research studies.

Chapter 6 examines the use of mixed methods and methodologies in research. It introduces the key ideas in evaluation research and the nature, scope and practice of action research in nursing, including data collection methods. This chapter establishes that there is often a need to employ mixed methodologies and methods in healthcare research in order to gain a more holistic view of some of the complex issues that surround the provision of nursing care.

The final short chapter, Chapter 7, considers how the thoughtful use of research can inform both what you do as a student nurse in practice and how research might be assimilated into your academic work to add to its depth and credibility. It demonstrates that research is not a dry academic topic but one potential source of increased knowledge to guide thinking and nursing practice.

NMC Standards of Proficiency

This edition refers to the Nursing and Midwifery Council's *Future Nurse: Standards of Proficiency for Registered Nurses* (NMC, 2018a) as they pertain to your development as a nurse, although its content is not narrowly defined by these standards.

Learning features

Learning from reading text is not always easy. Therefore, to provide variety and to assist with the development of independent learning skills and the application of theory to practice, this book contains activities, case studies, concept summaries, further reading and useful websites to enable you to participate in your own learning. You will need to develop your own study skills and 'learn how to learn' to get the best from the material. The book cannot provide all the answers, but instead provides a framework for your learning.

The activities in the book will help you in particular to make sense of, and learn about, the material being presented. Some activities ask you to reflect on aspects of practice, or your experience of it, or the people or situations you encounter. *Reflection* is an essential skill in nursing, and it helps you to understand the world around you and often to identify how things might be improved. Other activities will help you develop key graduate skills such as your ability to *think critically* about a topic in order to challenge received wisdom, or your ability to *research a topic and find appropriate information and evidence*, and to be able to make decisions using that evidence in situations that are often difficult and time-pressured. Communication and working as part of a team are core to all nursing practice, and some activities will ask you to think about your *communication skills* to help develop these.

All the activities require you to take a break from reading the text, think through the issues presented and carry out some independent study, possibly using the internet. Where appropriate, sample answers are presented at the end of each chapter, and these will help you to understand more fully your own reflections and independent study. You will gain most from the activities if you try to complete them yourself before reading the suggested answers. Remember, academic study will always require independent work; attending lectures will never be enough to be successful in your programme, and these activities will help to deepen your knowledge and understanding of the issues under scrutiny and give you practice at working on your own.

You might want to think about completing these activities as part of your personal development plan (PDP) or portfolio. After completing an activity write it up in your PDP or portfolio in a section devoted to that particular skill, then look back at it over time to see how far you have developed. You can also do more of the activities for a particular key skill that you have identified as a weakness, which will help build your skill and confidence in this area.

There is a glossary of terms at the end of the book that provides an interpretation of some of the terminology in the context of the subject of the book. Glossary terms are in **bold** in the first instance that they appear.

All chapters have further reading and useful websites listed at the end, with notes to show you why we think they will be helpful to you. The websites will also help you to remain up to date with developments in this aspect of practice as awareness of key issues grows and policies develop.

This fifth edition of *Understanding Research for Nursing Students* has been updated and improved in response to feedback from the earlier editions. We hope that you find this book helpful in developing your professional practice and that it challenges you to ensure you provide care and support that reduces the risk of vulnerability and promotes dignity, respect and a positive quality of life. Good luck with your studies!

Chapter 1 Introducing research

Chapter aims

After reading this chapter, you will be able to:

- describe the nature of research in health and social care;
- describe the type of questions that health and social care research is used to address;
- demonstrate awareness of the philosophical underpinning of research;
- identify the ethical considerations that need to be taken account of in research.

Introduction

The human condition is such that we are always striving to better ourselves and our lives. This is especially true of our health and the care we give and receive; certainly, considerable sums are spent each year on research and development into health and healthcare provision. Many nurses think that research is something that is beyond them, something other people do, and what they should do is simply respond by adopting new working practices following critical appraisal of the research. Unfortunately, practical, political and ethical restrictions on the undertaking of research by undergraduate and pre-registration healthcare professionals mean this is, indeed, all too often the case, and many nurses will never have the opportunity to experience the wonder of being the first to understand something or of discovering a new truth.

The reality about people who do research in nursing is not that they are different or in some way better than other nurses, it is more the fact they have learned to ask questions about care and care provision. They have learned to ask questions in very specific ways, ways that allow for the question to be explored, and in some instances answered, in a meaningful way. The purpose of this book is to introduce you to the **methodologies** and **methods** nursing and other healthcare researchers use to explore the exciting and challenging world of care provision.

Let us consider for a moment what is meant by research in the context of this book. The term 'research' is used to describe the structured and conscious application of scientific method to the exploration of an issue of interest in order either to understand the issue better or to establish new truths. This process of understanding or establishing new truths is termed **empirical** research. Empiricism is about understanding the nature of reality and so empirical research is about discovering new knowledge and understandings.

Over the next five chapters, this book will examine the major methodologies, methods and analytical processes used in nursing research. The aim is to enable you not only to read and understand research in this area but also to think about how and why research is important to what we do as nurses. The book will establish what constitutes an appropriate research question, how research is undertaken, where and with whom research is undertaken and what it can reasonably answer. If you want to understand what evidence is and how to carry out **critical appraisal** in order for it to contribute to evidence-based practice, you should read *Evidence-Based Practice in Nursing*, also in this series (Ellis, 2019).

Some of the terminology used in this chapter will become more familiar and easier to understand the further you get into the book or your research module.

Concept summary: empiricism

The terms empirical and empiricism refer to a way of knowing the world through the use of the senses. Empirical enquiry is about using observable, measurable and recordable ways of justifying what we do. Empirical enquiry uses: systematic observation; interviews; surveys; psychological testing; clinical testing and other types of examination. The emphasis in empiricism is therefore that all ideas (**hypotheses** and **theories**; see pages 83 and 87) have to be tested by observation and cannot be proven purely by reason or reflection. So the way in which research and the research process are structured is strongly influenced by the philosophy which underpins empiricism; that is, we can only know what we can observe. It is important to be aware that our ability to observe depends on the current state of science, which changes over time. For example, we now have MRI and CT scanning, which means we can see things we previously could not, and what we know about the human body has changed as a result. This does mean that what *we know*, or more correctly think we know, changes over time.

The research process

Coming up with a research question and then designing, undertaking, analysing and reporting research is a structured procedure that almost invariably follows the same process (see the box, 'The stages of the research process'). The **research process** ensures the research undertaken is fit for purpose; that is, it addresses the issue under consideration in a methodical manner.

The stages of the research process

- identification of the issue in need of research (often a clinical issue);
- undertaking a literature review (this stage is omitted in some qualitative methodologies);
- stating the purpose of the research (what it is trying to achieve);
- deciding the specific research questions, aims, objectives or hypotheses;
- collecting the data;
- analysing and interpreting the data;
- evaluating and reporting the research findings.

The identification of a topic for research will usually be a response to a clinical or practice-related requirement. Such questions might arise out of uncertainty about what to do or what might work best for a given situation. In turn this uncertainty leads the researcher to the need to review the existing literature in a given area with the purpose of deciding what it is the research can reasonably be expected to answer (dependent on the nature of the question being asked; see research paradigms on page 14). Sometimes a review of the literature will identify that there is no need to undertake research in order to answer the practice question, because the question has already been adequately answered.

If the question has not been answered before, then the nature of the problem being addressed will determine the way in which the research question is asked. Since different research methodologies and methods are used to answer different types of research questions, data collection will be determined not by researcher preference but by the need to use the right methodology and methods. For example, if a question is about the handwashing *behaviours* of staff, the data collection methodology will need to include some element of observation (because we can observe behaviour), while if the question relates to staff *understanding* the need for handwashing, then staff understanding can only be measured using questionnaires or interviews (because we have to ask people about their understanding).

Once collected, the analysis of data needs to be driven by the type of data collected for the study, so data in numerical form (numbers) will require statistical analysis and those in word form will need some form of data analysis, which involves analysing words. All research should then be subjected to some consideration of how well it has answered the original research question: Was it able to answer the question? Were there issues with the process that might be improved?

All these elements of the research process will be addressed in more detail in subsequent sections of this chapter and in more specific detail within the various chapters of this book.

The uncertainty principle

The starting point for all research is uncertainty. It is the lack of certainty in an area that creates a question. Uncertainty arises in all areas of health and social care, from questioning whether a new drug will cure cancer to understanding what it is like to live with respiratory disease.

Concept summary: the uncertainty principle

The **uncertainty principle** is the starting point for all research, as it establishes that there is something about the care we provide that we are not sure of. We may be uncertain how

(Continued)

(Continued)

patients make sense of living with a disease, or how they understand the care we are provid-ing, or indeed whether the care we provide is beneficial to them. Uncertainty causes us to ask questions. If we take the examples above and apply them to specific care scenarios, some questions we might ask are:

- What is it like to live with multiple sclerosis?
- Do patients undergoing chemotherapy understand its purpose?
- Does daily dressing of pressure ulcers aid their healing?
- What are the mental health issues facing individuals with learning disabilities?

Each of these scenarios is important in different ways, and each leads us to ask questions about what we do as nurses; each also contains an element of uncertainty.

If the starting point for research is uncertainty, where do we go next? Plainly there is a need to frame research questions that are relevant to the problem being consid-ered and able to address the uncertainty raised. Notably, because of the element of uncertainty that underlies each question, there is also uncertainty about whether the question we pose can be answered satisfactorily. So at the heart of research lies uncer-tainty not only about an element of care but also about how, and whether, we can answer the questions raised. Research seeks to answer questions, but there are no guar-antees it can; in fact, much research never adequately answers the big questions but goes some way towards answering some aspects of a topic or answering the question as it applies in one place and at one point in time.

Think of it like this. At election time we gain a snapshot of how some citizens of a country, those who vote, feel about the policies of the different political parties, in as much as people understand them. Even this snapshot is affected by one or two key issues (like the economy or immigration); how popular an individual politician is; and the way some people always vote for the same party every time. We know political parties come into power and leave power, therefore the ways in which these factors interact change over time, so we can never answer the question of which political party is most popular because the answer only applies at one point in time and in relation to who actually votes.

Why is research important then? Why do it, if we cannot guarantee it will answer our questions? These are reasonable concerns. Any research is only as good as the meth-odologies and methods it employs. All research methodologies and methods have strengths and weaknesses, and all research findings are open to being disproved or modified by later research. What is important about nursing research is that research-ers try, to the best of their ability, to answer important questions about the care we give informed by our current understandings and research abilities.

Using research to answer questions about the care we give is important because it allows us to develop increasing certainty about what we do. It allows us, as nurses, to be able to justify our practice; it provides, at least in part, an evidence base. Of course there are some questions which cannot be answered by research because of practical, financial or ethical constraints.

Activity 1.1   Critical thinking

Thinking about yourself or your family, why might you want the care that you might receive to be based on research evidence?

There are some possible answers to all activities at the end of the chapter, unless otherwise indicated.

Developing research questions

So far we have seen that the starting point for research is uncertainty about a question or questions that arise out of clinical practice. How, then, do we ask questions and what structures might we apply to the process?

Asking questions for research requires considerable thought, not only about the question itself but about whether the answer already exists. It may be that the questions arise out of clinical observations or interactions that have occurred in practice. Such questions may lead us down one of two pathways. The first is to seek clarification of the state of knowledge by reading the existing literature; the second is to ask questions that as yet have no, or only limited, answers.

Reviewing the literature on a topic is itself a skill and one with which you may already be familiar. Online bibliographic databases, such as the Cumulative Index of Nursing and Allied Health Literature (CINAHL), are a first point of call for many researchers. It is worth making the effort to learn and understand the processes by which these databases can be searched. Your university or hospital librarian will be able to help with this.

It is important to realise that, even if research has already been carried out within a given area, there may still be questions about its usefulness. For example, the National Institute for Health and Care Excellence (NICE), which reviews the evidence for clinical treatments in England, asks within its process and methods guide (2015) whether uncertainties apply to the use of research because of issues like applicability of the research to a specific group of people.

For instance, because a particular health education programme has worked in England for older people with hypertension, it will not necessarily work with younger people or among people who have another disease. The applicability of a study to other people and other places is a measure of its **external validity** (Fink, 2019), also known as its **generalisability**.

The Care Quality Commission (CQC), in a report into how the use of resources in NHS trusts are assessed (2015), makes the important point that the effective use of resources is necessary to ensure delivery of sustainable high-quality care. This underlines the point that some interventions in the health and social care setting may be so expensive and their benefits so minimal that it may not be appropriate to use them. Indeed, we may, in the process of reviewing the literature, identify other, less costly, interventions that provide a similar, or equal, level of benefit. Clearly, there are also ethical questions about what level and types of healthcare interventions society should fund.

NICE undertakes appraisals of clinical evidence to inform practice and ensure NHS money is used wisely. For example, NICE's (2018) *NICE Impact: Cancer* report claims to:

> *assess the clinical- and cost-effectiveness of new medicines, significant licence extensions and other health technologies. This is to ensure that all NHS patients have equitable access to the most clinically- and cost-effective treatments that are available.*

This statement demonstrates that:

- the clinical effectiveness of a product or process is assessed;
- the cost-effectiveness of the product or process is assessed;
- access to the process or product is equitable (i.e. ethically fair).

Questions about benefit, cost and ethics must be asked of any intervention to ensure its fitness for clinical application.

Gaining answers to these distinct, but interrelated, questions is important both when searching the literature and in planning research. Having answers to all of these questions helps would-be researchers decide whether what they want to do is of potential benefit.

Once the research literature has been searched and a need for further research identified, the researcher will move on to formulating a question that will guide the design and execution of the research project.

Two models for question formulation are widely used in health and social research. These models allow the researcher to focus not only on the research question but also on how the literature databases will be searched. Each model employs an acronym (SPICE and PICO) that helps the researcher focus and frame the research question in a logical and methodical manner.

The SPICE model is commonly applied to research aimed at answering qualitative questions. SPICE stands for:

- Setting
- Perspective
- Intervention

- Comparison
- Evaluation.

A couple of examples of the application of the SPICE model will illustrate how it helps to frame the search and research question. In our first example, we want to explore patients' understanding of living with asthma:

- We choose to focus on patients who are not usually unwell as a result of their asthma, and so concentrate on the general practice *setting*.
- The *perspective* of the study, that is, what the research is about, is clearly asthma, and perhaps more precisely the participants' understandings (perspective) of living with asthma. Because we are interested in people's understanding, we will not be applying an *intervention*.
- *Comparisons* of understanding might arise, possibly by chance, from the study – for instance between those newly diagnosed and those with a long-established diagnosis.
- The *evaluation* of the study will involve understanding people's perceptions of living with asthma and exploring these perceptions.

Activity 1.2   Critical thinking

Using the SPICE model, decide how you might frame a research question relating to a problem or issue from your area of practice. Remember, it is not necessary to use all the elements of the models in every type of research. Which of the elements you use will depend on the type of question you are asking.

As the answer is based on your own observation, there is no outline answer at the end of the chapter.

In our second example we are interested in the effects of an education programme on people's understanding of living with asthma:

- Our *setting* is again general practice.
- Our *perspective* remains the participants' understanding of living with asthma.
- Because we want to measure the effects of the education programme, we are clearly applying an *intervention*, which is the education programme.
- In order to demonstrate the effectiveness of the programme, or not, we need something to *compare* it to. This might be people's understanding of living with asthma before and then after the programme, or it might be the difference in understanding between one group who had the intervention and another group who did not.
- Our *evaluation* will then consist of identifying the level of difference in understanding before and after the education programme, either for the individual or between the intervention and non-intervention groups.

The PICO model is usually applied to research studies that involve an intervention, although, as we have seen, the SPICE model can also be used for this purpose. PICO stands for:

- Patient or Problem
- Intervention
- Comparison
- Outcome.

PICO will work equally well as a method of illuminating the elements of the second example above:

- In this instance, therefore, *patient* refers to patients in general practice with asthma.
- The *intervention* remains the education programme.
- *Comparison* is still that of understanding before and after the education programme.
- *Outcome* refers to the improvement, or not, in patients' understanding of living with asthma.

Activity 1.3 Critical thinking

Using the PICO model, decide how you might frame a research question relating to a problem or issue from your area of practice. Remember, it is not necessary to use all of the elements of the models in every type of research. Which of the elements you use will depend on the type of question you are asking.

As the answer is based on your own observation, there is no outline answer at the end of the chapter.

Once framed in this way, it is easier to create a list of all the words and phrases associated with the potential research question. This list will itself enable you to structure your literature review, which will in turn inform the research plan. Such a list will include not only the key words but also synonyms, as well as lay and technical terminology. For example, pressure ulcers may appear as pressure sores, decubitus ulcers, bed sores and skin ulcers. It would be useful to search using all these terms.

It is also helpful to apply some limits within which the bibliographic database should search – for example, it may be helpful to limit the search to the last five or ten years depending on the topic. It is also worth asking your hospital or university librarian about access to other sources of information such as unpublished reports or university theses.

The literature search and identification of existing research are likely to leave you in one of three positions. The first is that the topic that you are interested in has already been well researched, and the research covers a similar patient group to the one you care for. Depending on the age of the research, you may feel further research to inform a potential change in practice is unnecessary. However, it is always worth being cautious about applying research that has only been undertaken once without putting in place some form of local evaluation and audit of the change. This is because sometimes research can actually come to the wrong conclusions!

The second position is that the research has been done, but in a group, or in a place, very dissimilar to where you want to apply it. For example, the research may have been done abroad, the ages of the participants may be very different from the patients that you care for, or the patients may have come from a different ethnic or cultural background. That is, the external validity, or generalisability, of the research does not extend to the patients you are caring for.

The third situation is that the research has not been done anywhere you can find. So you are left where you started, with a question or questions that need answering. It is important to look at these questions and identify approaches that might usefully be employed in answering them. At this point, it might be useful to return to your PICO or SPICE model to help you think about how to structure and present the research question.

Activity 1.4   Research and finding out

As well as the SPICE and PICO models, a number of other models exist to aid in question formulation. These include PEO, CLIP, ECLIPSE and SPIDER. Go online and search for tools for developing research questions and see what you can find. For each model you identify, write at least one research question. For a good starting point see useful websites at the end of the chapter.

As the answer is based on your own observation, there is no outline answer at the end of the chapter.

Before we go on to explore how we place our question within a research framework, a note of caution is needed. Some research, such as grounded theory and phenomenology (explained in Chapter 2), requires researchers to start with limited preconceptions about what they might find. This means it may be necessary for a researcher to avoid engaging in a full literature search at the start of the study. This is something that should be discussed with a research supervisor.

Good research questions will summarise the key elements the research will address; they indicate the type of information the person posing the question wants. You may have noticed the questions we have asked so far fall into two distinct categories. The first category includes questions about things we can measure directly, such as the rate of healing of a pressure ulcer. The second category is about feelings, understanding and being, and is therefore more difficult to measure in any direct, objective way.

Research paradigms

This difference in the emphasis of the questions asked leads us to the first rung of the research ladder: identifying the nature of the question being asked. In research terminology this means we need to identify the **paradigm** within which the question sits. Simply put, paradigms are the philosophical basis of the question being asked; the nature of the enquiry needed in order to address the question that has been identified.

In health and social care research, as in most practical research, it is usual to identify two paradigms, the **quantitative paradigm** and the **qualitative paradigm**. These refer to different ways of viewing the world and reality.

The quantitative paradigm is the one you might most associate with scientific ways of thinking. It involves viewing the world in ways that are measurable (or provable). The 'quantitative' element of the paradigm refers to the ability of research within this paradigm to quantify its findings. In other words, the findings can be counted or can be demonstrated in a way that is measurable.

Quantitative research is concerned with proof, with cause and effect and with demonstrating associations between **variables**. It often starts with a hypothesis, an idea yet to be tested using established scientific methods. Chapter 4 explores the approaches that lie within this research paradigm.

Activity 1.5   Reflection

Given that the quantitative research paradigm is concerned with things that can be counted, and with cause and effect, think about what questions you could ask in your work setting. What clinical problems might be best answered using this approach?

Keep your notes on this safe and return to them when you read Chapter 4, where you will find examples of this type of research to compare them with.

Data collection within the quantitative paradigm is often **deductive**. That is, quantitative research usually starts with a hypothesis, or idea, that it seeks to confirm or refute. Deductive reasoning follows predetermined methods for collecting data. Deductive research works from general observations towards a more specific outcome and in this respect it is considered to be knowledge-driven – that is, it is about things we think we know, such as things we see and things we can quantify. Its primary purpose is to prove or disprove areas of perceived knowledge. Figure 1.1 gives a diagrammatic representation of deductive research.

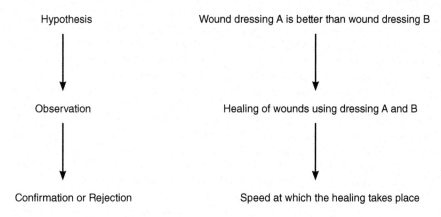

Figure 1.1 Representation of deductive research

The qualitative paradigm is the one that you might most associate with the social sciences and 'people-centred' methods of enquiry. It is a way of looking at the world from the point of view of people. It enquires about what people experience, feel, think, understand and believe. The qualitative paradigm is not so concerned with proof – more with describing and understanding human experiences from the point of view of the people who have had, or are having, the experience.

The 'qualitative' element of the paradigm refers to the fact that it seeks to understand things that cannot readily be measured or counted. It is more concerned with the quality of an experience and of understanding and belief. Qualitative research starts with a question, something that needs to be explored; it may be used to generate a hypothesis or theory (as in the methodology called **grounded theory**), but it does not start with one. Chapter 2 explores the approaches to enquiry used within this paradigm.

Activity 1.6   Reflection

Given that the qualitative research paradigm is concerned with things that cannot be counted, such as human experiences and understanding, think about what questions you could ask about where you currently work that fit this paradigm. What clinical problems might be best answered using this approach?

Keep your notes on this safe and return to them in Chapter 2, where you will find examples of this type of research to which you can compare your answer.

Qualitative research is by nature **inductive**, that is, it generates ideas and theories from what is observed. The data collected lead to the generation of ideas or hypotheses

(hypotheses tested in deductive studies are sometimes derived from inductive research). The researchers start out on an enquiry not knowing what they will find; they allow the data collected to lead them to the creation of a new idea or hypothesis. Inductive research works from specific observations towards creating much broader generalisations. Sometimes described as 'feature detecting', qualitative research methodologies use observations and interviews to detect the key features of a phenomenon. Figure 1.2 gives a diagrammatic representation of inductive research.

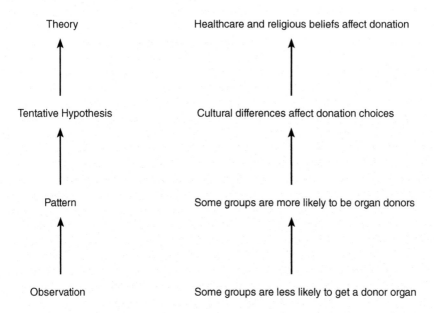

Figure 1.2 Representation of inductive research

It is worth reflecting on the education proficiency introduced at the start of this chapter that requires nurses to 'demonstrate an understanding of research methods, ethics and governance in order to critically analyse, safely use, share and apply research findings to promote and inform best nursing practice'.

This assumes an understanding of the theoretical basis of research and the variety of questions research can be used to answer. We have established that there are two key routes to understanding the world of healthcare using the qualitative and quantitative paradigms. Now it is important we identify how these apparently opposing world views are used to answer research questions arising in the clinical setting.

Within each paradigm, a number of approaches to research are used to answer specific types of questions. These approaches are called research methodologies. The following section introduces you to the key elements of the research methodologies that will be explored in more depth in Chapters 2 and 4.

It is important to note at this stage that stating there are two approaches to research is an artificial construct: the world is complex and most issues that affect humans require a broader understanding which requires not only that we understand how something, say a drug, works (quantitative) but also how people experience the effects and side effects of the drug and how it makes them feel (qualitative). Chapter 6 explores the overlap in these paradigms and their associated methodologies and methods.

Research methodologies

If the research paradigms are the schools of thought upon which research is based, the methodologies represent the more detailed plan of action (the blueprint) used to execute the research. Methodologies supply structure to the research process as they are designed to be undertaken in specific ways in order to answer specific questions.

Examples of the use of a methodology within a paradigm include **randomised controlled trials**, which seek to prove cause and effect and so sit within the quantitative paradigm, and **phenomenology**, which explores people's lived experiences of a phenomenon and sits within the qualitative paradigm. Table 1.1 shows the research paradigms and the major research methodologies explored in this book. This is not an exhaustive list, and, as we shall see at various points in the book, clinical questions often generate the need for research to operate in more than one paradigm.

Research paradigm	Qualitative paradigm	Quantitative paradigm
Research methodologies	Phenomenology	Randomised controlled trial
	Grounded theory	Cohort study
	Ethnography	Case-control studies
	Case study	Cross-sectional studies

Table 1.1   The research paradigms and their major associated methodologies

Research methodologies are, therefore, the overall scheme by which research is undertaken, and the choice of methodology is driven by the nature of the research question being asked.

We now know that the broad research question determines the paradigm within which a research approach lies and that the specific question will then determine the methodology to be applied. Other factors influence the choice of methodology used to answer a specific research question. These include practical and ethical issues as well as looking at the types of question a methodology can answer. Chapters 2 and 4 will examine in more detail how the choice to use a particular methodology is made and why.

Although not strictly a research methodology, literature reviews are a means of generating new understandings from existing research in order to inform practice. There are a number of ways in which previously published research can be examined either to inform practice directly, or in the design and undertaking of subsequent research.

At one end are the incomplete narrative-type reviews a student might undertake to inform the writing of an essay; this involves some searching of a topic using a bibliographic database and the indiscriminate use of the findings as references. At the other end are **systematic reviews** of the literature which attempt to identify all the research published about a topic within a chosen timeframe. The data from the identified research are then evaluated for quality and used to write a review with a state-of-the-art understanding of the topic. The process by which research that is included in the review is evaluated is strictly defined and adhered to and is explained as part of the process of writing up the review. Sometimes systematic reviews include **meta-analyses** (when the data used in the analyses of each study within a systematic review are collated and reanalysed as if they were one large dataset).

Whatever you are reading research for, there is always a need to appraise it critically for the quality of the research process, as this ultimately impacts on the level of faith you can place in the findings – and therefore whether or not you wish to apply them in your own workplace. Critical appraisal is a structured and thoughtful process whereby the quality of a piece of research is assessed using agreed criteria in order to establish its quality and applicability to your own practice. Critical appraisal is covered in some detail, along with some tools for applying the process to different research paradigms, in *Evidence-Based Practice in Nursing,* also in this series (Ellis, 2019).

Research methods

Research methods are the tools, the practical equipment, by which the information for an enquiry is collected. The choice of paradigm and subsequent research methodology will determine which research methods are used in an enquiry.

The methods of data collection have to fit the type of question asked. For example, if the research is about understanding how people feel, how they see the world or how they see their experiences, then the researcher needs to ask them about these things. Such an enquiry requires the researcher to engage in dialogue with the research subjects, using interviews and focus groups in order to gain an insight into their world. These issues cannot be measured or quantified in any meaningful way, so these qualitative methods allow an insight into someone else's world that cannot be gained using quantitative methods.

Conversely, it is not possible to demonstrate that a new wound dressing has additional clinical benefit for patients by talking to them. Such things need to be measured, and the new dressing and an existing dressing need to be compared. In order to undertake such an enquiry, the researcher will need to take biological and clinical measurements that can be enumerated. For example, how long does this type of wound take to heal? How many days does the patient spend in hospital? What percentage of people in whom this type of dressing is used, for this type of wound, develop an infection? These questions cannot be addressed meaningfully, or accurately, by qualitative methodologies;

although it is fair to say that patients should be asked about their experience of the dressing, its comfort and tolerability.

A researcher also needs to take into account other considerations when designing and undertaking a study. Some of these will be explored in the following sections.

Activity 1.7   Research and finding out

Before reading the rest of the chapter, make some notes about what other things a researcher might need to take into account when designing a study. Perhaps take the idea of a wound dressing as a prompt for your deliberations.

An outline of what you might find is given at the end of the chapter.

Ethical considerations in research

Ethics permeate all we do in the delivery of health and social care. It is a requirement of nursing practice that we act in ways that are ethical and take into account the rights of the people we care for (see the Nursing and Midwifery Council's (NMC) *Code*, 2018b). Ethical considerations in research are important for many reasons, not least of which is that people enter into research studies of their own free will (unlike entering hospital when unwell, for example) and that the research we are undertaking is premised on the uncertainty principle.

It is a sad fact that some of the clinical information we use today in healthcare provision has been obtained at the expense of the weak and vulnerable. Examples that spring to mind are the atrocities committed by Nazi doctors in the name of medical research in the concentration and extermination camps of the Second World War. But there are many more recent examples of unethical and immoral practices in healthcare within societies considered to be world leaders in the promotion and protection of human rights.

Case study

The Tuskegee Study of Untreated Syphilis in the Negro Male was a clinical study of the effects of syphilis conducted over the 40 years between 1932 and 1972 in Tuskegee, Alabama, in the USA. A total of 399 male African Americans infected with syphilis were enrolled in the study along with a control group of 201 (people without syphilis). All of the

(Continued)

(Continued)

participants were poor, most were illiterate and they did not give informed consent. They were not told about their diagnosis; rather, they were told they had 'bad blood' and would get taken to the clinic to receive free medical treatment, as well as free meals and burial insurance, as incentives for participating.

When the study started, existing treatments for syphilis were often toxic and of limited, if any, effectiveness. One of the initial aims of the study was to establish whether patients were better off not being treated with these dubious remedies. Many participants were therefore denied any treatment, and others were lied to and given placebo (fake) treatments so that the fatal progression of the syphilis could be observed.

Many participants died of syphilis, or related complications. Some wives were also infected during the study and gave birth to children with syphilis. From 1947 it had been known that syphilis could be effectively treated with penicillin.

The Declaration of Helsinki

Such instances, as well as other notoriously unethically conducted studies, led to the establishment of various conventions and international agreements on the ethical conduct of research involving human subjects. Perhaps the most widely known of these is the Declaration of Helsinki, first published by the World Medical Association in 1964 and most recently revised in 2013 (WMA, 2013). There are three key tenets of the Declaration of Helsinki:

1. Studies should be of a generally acceptable scientific standard.
2. The study should cause no harm.
3. The study subjects should have given their full consent.

What this means for the various stages of the research process depends upon interpretation and the type of research being undertaken. Before exploring in a little more detail the application of ethics to research, it is worth considering what approaches to ethics might be used to inform that process.

Activity 1.8   Research and finding out

Before reading the rest of the chapter, go online and find the Declaration of Helsinki and familiarise yourself with some of its principles.

The URL for the website is in the further reading section at the end of the chapter.

Approaches to ethics

Beauchamp and Childress (2013) present the ethical principles of **beneficence** (doing good), **non-maleficence** (doing no harm), **autonomy** (respecting choice) and **justice** (fairness) as one way of viewing the moral and ethical obligations of human beings. These principles may equally well be applied to research being undertaken in the human setting.

These are duty-based ethical principles that identify the individual human being as the central point of importance in ethical thinking and dictate the way in which researchers should behave towards their study participants. This duty-based (or **non-consequentialist**) approach requires researchers to follow certain rules of conduct regardless of their consequences. This way of thinking about ethics has strong associations with both Judaism and Christianity, as it is based on the standards of human behaviour dictated by the Ten Commandments.

In contrast to duty-based ethics, **utilitarian** (or **consequentialist**) **ethics** takes the view that the ends justify the means – that is, the consequence of the action is more important than the action undertaken. So, consequentialist ethics requires us to make a judgement about the likely outcome of a course of action, whereas duty-based ethics requires us always to act in a way that is in itself good.

We have seen that uncertainty is the starting point for all research, and so it might seem impossible to apply these principles to the research process precisely because we cannot be certain how the research will proceed and what its consequences might be. It is important, however, to take the view that ethics is as much about intentions as about what actually happens. If we accept that health and social care research is done with the best of intentions, and that some of the basic principles of ethics, such as avoiding *unnecessary* harm and aiming for a *good* outcome, are followed, it is possible to undertake research in an ethical way.

For the researcher setting out to undertake an enquiry, and for practising nurses reading the results of the research and seeking to use them in their day-to-day practice, it is important that the ethics of each stage of the research process is well established. Most, if not all, nursing, medical and health journals now require that research papers submitted for publication can show they have received ethics committee approval.

Ethics in the stages of research

Deciding what we are going to research and how raises ethical questions, including whether the potential benefits of the study are great enough to justify the time, money and effort that will be used in undertaking it. Because we cannot know for certain the answers to any of these issues, we have to ask questions about the intentions of the study. If the intention of the study is to improve the lives of future patients and clients, then it is reasonable to move to the next question.

Secondly, will the study inflict harm on the research subjects? Even qualitative enquiries, which involve little more than an interview or a focus group discussion, have the potential to upset people – for example, by encouraging them to confront thoughts and feelings they had suppressed. It is important, therefore, that if the effects of the study cannot be known before the study starts, there should at least be mechanisms in place to minimise any harm that does arise. In a qualitative study this might mean providing counselling or support services for participants. Making such provisions satisfies the requirements of avoiding deliberate harm as well as attaining the best consequences for research participants by minimising unforeseen and unintended consequences of the study.

If the study is likely to inflict some harm, as may be the case in a drug trial or a study of a new surgical procedure, we may wish to ask whether or not the likely outcomes of the study make the potential for harm worthwhile. All research must be designed in a way that minimises the likelihood of harm occurring – and be of a generally acceptable scientific standard (WMA, 2013). Any risks, or potential risks, associated with a study need to be disclosed at the point of gaining consent, so that whether the risk is worth taking is a decision that potential participants can make for themselves. The important thing about decisions people make with regard to being involved in research is therefore not whether they know what the outcome will be for them per se, but that they understand the potential risks and benefits and consent to accepting these.

Service user involvement

There is an increasing body of evidence demonstrating that the inclusion of lay members in the design and undertaking of research studies adds value to the studies' design and execution (National Institute for Health Research, 2013). Much health and social care research is about people and their understandings and experiences of care; it makes sense therefore that people who experience care are involved in the ways in which the quality and experience of care are measured.

McLaughlin (2008) identifies four levels of service user participation in research:

1. objects of research to be measured, used and then discarded;
2. at the foreground able to tell their story, although this is still tempered by the researcher;
3. having the ability to act and change and not seen as merely parts of the system;
4. acting as creators and co-creators of knowledge and understanding.

Increasingly it is the last sense of participation that is finding favour in health and social care research. One of the ethical tensions of research has often been that the people who commit the most to it – for example, taking a new medication or giving up their story of a particular experience – are those with the least control over the process, the research participants. Including at least some of the potential participants of the research in its design, undertaking, analysis and writing up makes the process more inclusive and demonstrates a commitment to seeing people as equal partners in the process rather than objects on which to do research.

Gaining consent

The gaining and maintenance of consent are regarded as an ongoing process, not a one-off event, by the Health Research Authority (HRA, 2014) and the NMC (2018b). Gaining valid consent for any study may appear impossible given that the outcome of the research is not known at the point that the consent is gained! This should not impede the process of research, nor should it be thought that it makes the process of gaining consent fraudulent. Consent gained in relation to a piece of research is for the participation of the individual in a process that will lead to an (as yet uncertain) outcome. Consent to participate in research has to be obtained in all cases and for all types of studies.

Gaining consent takes into account a number of separate elements:

- the **mental capacity** and **competence** of the potential participant to give consent;
- the understanding of the information given;
- freedom from **coercion**;
- freedom of choice;
- the understanding of the right to withdraw.

Given the nature of health and social care research, research participants are likely to be in some way vulnerable (e.g. in poor health or elderly). This vulnerability leads to concerns about the capacity and competence of the individuals to consent (Biros, 2018). Such concerns include people who, when well, are undoubtedly competent.

It is clear that some individuals are not, and will never be, competent to give consent – for example, people with dementia and young children. In the UK the HRA provides clear guidance on what to do in situations where the consent of an individual cannot be gained because of that person's age or illness. This includes respecting previously given consent, or withheld consent, and seeking the consent of the next of kin or parents where appropriate (HRA, 2014).

Next, we must ensure that potential research participants for a study have received information about the study and understood it. This means producing information sheets written in a manner potential participants can understand, checking potential participants have understood and explaining any ambiguities or misunderstandings. It is at this stage that the help of lay collaborators in research can be invaluable. While understanding is in some respects affected by competence and capacity, the test of good information giving is that the people at whom the information is aimed can, on the whole, understand it.

Freedom from coercion means ensuring that potential participants do not feel under any obligation to take part in the study. Coercion may result from the fact that the potential participant and the researcher are in a dependent relationship, including nurse–patient or student–lecturer relationships. In such cases, great care must be taken to ensure that potential research participants are aware that they are under no obligation to take part, and that not taking part will have no adverse effect on their care or education. One way this is often achieved is by using a third party to recruit research participants.

Freedom of choice means ensuring potential participants understand they are under no obligation to choose to take part in the study. The choice made should be one they enter into, having read and understood the information given to them and decided they want to participate. They must be free to choose not to participate if that is their wish. It is usual to see statements like: 'Whether or not you decide to take part in the study, your care will not be affected'.

Research participants should also understand they have the right to withdraw from a study at any point. This is what is meant by consent being an ongoing process. Just because individuals agree to start a study does not mean that they have to see it through to the end against their wishes.

Confidentiality

A further key element of research ethics is the protection of the confidentiality of research participants. All participants in any study have the right to expect that they will not be identifiable when the findings of the research are made public, and that participation in research will not in any way disadvantage them. The advent of genetic diagnoses has made the issue of participant data confidentiality very topical. Participants are worried that data taken from their DNA for research purposes could lead to increased insurance premiums if the data suggest that they have a high risk of developing a genetically determined disease.

Aside from these 'high-tech' studies, people involved in studies in which they express controversial opinions or disclose personal information about their battle with disease may wish for the source of this information to be kept private. It is therefore incumbent on the ethical researcher to adhere to a strict code of confidentiality both while undertaking the research and when writing it up for publication or conference presentation.

That all said, there is an ever-present tension for the nurse researcher who may, during the course of their research, uncover practices or behaviours which threaten the safety of patients. In other instances, the participant may disclose that they are engaged in illegal practices or that they intend harming themselves (Leyva-Moral and Feijoo-Cid, 2017). Such cases create moral dilemmas for researchers whose duty may be to break the code of confidentiality usually associated with research.

Activity 1.9   Reflection

Consider your time in practice and the occasions when you have been privy to confidential information. Consider and reflect on those occasions when you have felt conflicted about keeping a confidence and what reasons gave rise to your dilemma. Discuss your thoughts with your practice supervisor and try to gain a better understanding of how you might manage difficult situations with regard to confidentiality in the future.

As this activity is based on your own reflection, there is no specimen answer at the end of the chapter.

Disseminating research

At the start of the research process we saw how important it was to look into the existing literature in order either to inform an immediate change in practice or to design a research study. This means that there is an ethical requirement for researchers to make the findings of their work public. Withholding the findings of research has consequences for other researchers, who may set out to undertake research into an area that has already been explored, using time and money that could be better spent elsewhere. It also means that the lessons which might have been learned, and subsequently applied to practice, have not been.

There are a number of reasons why not all studies get published. Sometimes the research is undertaken as part of a course of study, and students, on getting their award, feel that they have completed all they need to do. Sometimes the research comes out with a result that was unexpected – it disproves the hypothesis, perhaps. This may lead some researchers not to publish, especially where the research has been sponsored by an organisation that may be damaged by negative findings. Another reason research with negative findings does not get published is that it is rejected by publishers because it does not make good reading – this is known as publication **bias**.

If we return to our guiding ethical principles, we can say that not publishing or making the findings of research known is potentially unethical for two reasons: it may inflict harm on others and it may lead to negative consequences. The 'others' on whom harm may be inflicted include:

- people who volunteered for the study who expected their sacrifice to benefit other people;
- researchers who subsequently design studies that are in the same area or contain the same flaws that might have been identified if they had seen the previous research;
- current patients who may be subjected to care that research has shown does not work or could be better in some material way;
- society at large, which may be spending tax money on substandard care.

Other issues to take into account when designing a research project

Even the simplest study will have some cost attached to it. Interviewing participants for a study may involve travel, the cost of the recording device and often the cost of professional transcription of the interview tapes. Other costs that may need to be considered, depending on the study, are postage, printing, and paperwork and telephone costs. Many novice researchers underestimate the time a study will take to do and so may not cost out the time away from work that research grants are often designed to help with.

The amount of time needed to undertake research often comes as a surprise to the first-time researcher. This will include the time taken to read textbooks regarding research design as well as the time taken to undertake a literature review of the topic under research. The study will then need to be written up for ethical and, potentially, research and development review (that is, a review of the scientific quality of the study as well as what the study may mean in terms of the use of facilities and staff time within the organisation within which it is set). It is necessary to write participant literature, undertake the data collection (whatever form that takes), review and analyse the data and then write the study up. Interestingly, the time taken to prepare to undertake the study and the time taken to analyse the findings are both often far in excess of the time taken to do the study itself.

Even the most experienced researchers will rely to some extent on the expertise of others at some stage of the research process – most commonly at the study design and analysis stages. It is often worth getting advice about how the study will be analysed (e.g. from a statistician) at the design stage in order to ensure that data that are collected are in the right format and of a type to allow for the best possible analysis. Collecting the correct type of data in the correct format is most important in quantitative studies that will be subjected to statistical analysis, as some forms of data will increase the power of the study.

Because a study can take a long time to do, one of the issues commonly affecting novice researchers is maintaining their interest, which can wane, especially during the design and analysis stages. One of the questions researchers must ask themselves at the start of any study is, therefore, 'Will this study hold my attention for its duration?'

Chapter summary

This chapter has introduced you to the key elements that need to be considered when setting out to undertake a research project. It has identified that, in nursing, there are two

(Continued)

(Continued)

broad approaches to answering clinical questions. These approaches – the quantitative and qualitative paradigms – have distinct features and may be used to answer specific types of questions. The choice of research paradigm is determined by the type of question the research seeks to answer, and it is important this is understood from the start of the research process. We also identified that the quantitative/qualitative distinction is artificial, and that our understanding of the world (and especially of people) is more complex than one or other paradigm can examine on its own.

We have seen that the choice of paradigm and the nature of the research question then leads researchers to select an overall methodology – research approach – for their study. The methodology chosen determines the methods, or research tools, that the researcher will apply in undertaking the research. We have briefly introduced the concept of literature reviews as a form of research methodology which pulls together the findings from existing research in a structured way in order to understand better a topic or phenomenon of interest.

The need to apply ethical considerations to all stages of the research process has been discussed, and ethical theories used to illustrate why this is important. Ethical considerations have been identified as being more important than scientific considerations when designing a research project. We identified the increasing understanding of the important role that participants can play in the design and undertaking of a research study. We have also looked at some of the practical considerations potential researchers must take into account before starting out on a research project if time and money are to be spent wisely.

Activities: brief outline answers

Activity 1.1 Critical thinking (page 9)

There are several reasons why research is important in informing care:

- it shows that what we do is ethical – it does good or at least avoids doing harm;
- it shows that public money is being used wisely;
- it demonstrates that of the care is of clinical benefit;
- it responds to the need for governance;
- it establishes the professional credibility of the care.

Activity 1.7 Research and finding out (page 19)

What researchers might need to take into account when designing a study:

- their own expertise;
- money;
- the availability of time;
- ethical issues;
- access to research subjects;
- availability of support;
- how they define things for inclusion, e.g. a wound;
- the characteristics of people in the study.

Further reading

Ellis, P (2019) *Evidence-Based Practice in Nursing* (4th edn). London: Sage.

Chapter 1 especially identifies why evidence for practice is so important and what constitutes evidence.

Fink, A (2019) *Conducting Research Literature Reviews* (5th edn). London: Sage.

An excellent text on how to undertake reviews of literature.

Moule, P (2021) *Making Sense of Research in Nursing, Health and Social Care* (7th edn). London: Sage.

Chapters 1 and 2 establish the need for and nature of research in the caring professions.

Moule, P (2016) *Nursing Research: An Introduction* (3rd edn). London: Sage.

Chapters 1 and 2 provide insight into evidence and the sources of knowledge in nursing.

Parahoo, K (2014) *Nursing Research: Principles, Process and Issues* (3rd edn). London: Palgrave Macmillan.

Chapters 1 and 2 provide a good overview of the sources of and need for knowledge in nursing.

Topping, A (2015) The quantitative–qualitative continuum, in Gerrish, K and Lathlean, J (eds) *The Research Process in Nursing* (7th edn). Oxford: Wiley-Blackwell.

A useful discussion of the nature of knowledge and qualitative and quantitative research paradigms.

Useful websites

www.hra.nhs.uk/about-the-hra/our-committees/research-ethics-committees-recs UK NHS Research Ethics Committee's website.

www.rcn.org.uk/professional-development/research-and-innovation You can subscribe here to a free e-bulletin on nursing research.

https://information-specialists.leeds.ac.uk/information-specialists/search-concept-tools/ Provides an overview of tools for developing research questions.

https://jbi.global/about-jbi The home of the Joanna Briggs Institute research organisation, which has many evidence-based information tools.

www.wma.net/policies-post/wma-declaration-of-helsinki-ethical-principles-for-medical-research-involving-human-subjects/ The World Medical Associations site with the Declaration of Helsinki.

Chapter 2   Overview of qualitative methodologies

Chapter aims

After reading this chapter, you will be able to:

- identify the main qualitative research methodologies used in health and social care;
- describe the type of research questions the different qualitative research methodologies can be used to answer;
- demonstrate awareness of how samples are chosen for qualitative studies;
- briefly describe the key methods of data collection used in qualitative enquiry.

Introduction

In Chapter 1, it was established that qualitative research answers questions about people's attitudes, experiences and opinions. Qualitative research differs from quantitative research in the way it approaches research questions. The key is in the name: quantitative research is concerned with quantity so uses numbers; qualitative research is concerned with the nature and *quality* of individuals' experience. The data used in qualitative research are words and sometimes pictures. Qualitative research is expressive and people-centred – that is, it is focused on people's lived experiences, attitudes, opinions and feelings.

Nursing is often described as both an art and a science. It is the art of nursing that qualitative research best addresses, as it answers questions not about the science of what we do as nurses but about the art of human interaction. At the same time, qualitative research tries to understand something of the lives of the people we care for. Nursing is a people-centred discipline, and qualitative research has found favour among nursing academics and practitioners because of its ability to ask and answer questions about what it is like to be someone else, what it is like to experience care and how people in receipt of care view that care.

As Table 2.1 shows, different kinds of qualitative research look at different forms of human interaction.

Research methodology	Usages
Phenomenology	Studies a phenomenon or experience of interest
Grounded theory	Generates a theory about a social interaction
Ethnography	Studies groups and cultures
Case study	Explores a case or a number of cases of interest
Generic qualitative	Follows the methods but does not identify a methodology

Table 2.1 The main qualitative research methodologies used in nursing

Key characteristics of qualitative research

Qualitative research is used to answer some of the questions that quantitative research cannot. For instance, we cannot measure someone's emotions or attitudes using a ruler or a thermometer, therefore we cannot quantify them – try as we might to create scales that measure this sort of data. Many questions that need answering about nursing and healthcare are not related to numbers of patients treated, the speed of recovery, time spent in hospital or mortality rates. Questions such as 'How well do I feel I have been cared for?' or 'What is it like to be treated in this dialysis unit?' are more about the perceived quality of the care provided than the actual amount.

It is worth noting the importance of experience to users of health and social care services here. A report into the NHS complaints system (Clwyd and Hart, 2013) identified the things people most often complain about in relation to their NHS care as being:

- lack of information;
- lack of compassion;
- neglect of dignity and caring;
- staff attitudes;
- resources.

What this indicates is that resources, things which can be counted, feature as only one of the five things people find most important about their care experience. It may be reasonable to assume, therefore, that quality of care, and the quality of the care experience, is at least as important as, if not more important than, the delivery of care itself to most people.

Activity 2.1 Critical thinking

Next time you are working clinically, try asking one or more service users this simple question: 'What are the things which are important to you when you are using a health or social care service?' Make a note of the responses and spend some time reflecting on how the views reflected in the answers are the same as or different from your view and of the themes identified in the preceding list.

As the answer will be based on your experience, there is no outline answer at the end of the chapter.

What is clear is that different people experience the same phenomenon or event in different ways. You only have to look at how different people will represent an event in a court of law to see this. An understanding of how the care we give is experienced by those we care for will therefore be of benefit to nurses who are concerned with *how* they deliver care and improve our delivery of care.

The radically different emphases of qualitative and quantitative questions, and the fact they are both important to our understanding of care, means there are a large number of differences not only in the philosophy underpinning each paradigm but also in the research methodologies and methods they use to answer questions.

Some academics and researchers like to claim that one paradigm is more important, or indeed better, than the other. This view of research as being competitive in nature and differing in importance is really quite short-sighted. It is better to think about the two forms of research as being of equal importance, with the findings from one complementing and adding extra dimensions to the findings of the other (Topping, 2015).

Quite often quantitative research generates the need for an answer to a qualitative question. That is, sometimes we find out things by experiment or measurement that leave us with another, equally or more important, question. For example, Professor Sir Richard Doll, with others, famously demonstrated the link between smoking and lung cancer, using quantitative research, but people continue to smoke. An important question that arises from this for nursing practice in terms of a public health message is, therefore, 'Why do people smoke?' The answers to why people start smoking and continue to smoke can only realistically be gained from an insight into the motivations, understandings and stories of people who smoke. Qualitative research methodologies and methods are needed to gain this valuable understanding.

It is only if and when we can answer such important questions as 'Why do people smoke?' that we can address the next logical question, 'How can we stop people from smoking?' Of course, the answer to this question may partially lie within a quantitative question such as, 'Is using nicotine replacement therapy better than not using it in helping people to quit smoking?' Or we may need to ask a question such as 'What do people say about what causes them to continue smoking when they know it is harming them?' – a qualitative enquiry.

The various qualitative methodologies have evolved to answer quite specific questions using often well-defined methods. For example, we will see that phenomenological research has developed to answer questions about the 'lived experience' or **essence** of a particular phenomenon, and the method usually used to answer this type of question is in-depth interviewing.

It is quite common for qualitative studies to identify themselves simply as 'a qualitative study' when published and not to identify one specific methodology that informed the approach to answering the question. While, in this chapter, specific qualitative research methodologies are presented as being used to answer specific questions using well-defined associated methods, it is reasonable for a qualitative researcher to adopt some of the methods of qualitative research in order to answer their research question without necessarily identifying and adopting a specific methodology and its associated philosophical and academic underpinnings.

This may seem odd. However, all experienced researchers know that in order to undertake any research successfully, compromises have to be made, and often established rules and conventions associated with a particular methodology may prove hard to follow in the pursuit of answering a specific question. The methods used and the processes adopted within the practice of qualitative research often evolve and develop during the life of the study (that is, the process is **iterative**) in response to difficulties encountered or insights gained. This evolution of methods and approaches is a practical response to the inductive nature of qualitative enquiry, which by its very nature is responsive to, and affected by, occurrences within the life of the study.

Concept summary: qualitative and quantitative differences

Both qualitative and quantitative researchers use similar data collection methods – such as interviews or observation. What differs between the two paradigms are what Sarantakos (2012) calls the *methodological standards*. For the quantitative researcher, interviews follow a rigid and reproducible structure, with the same questions asked in the same way to a large number of people to gain quantifiable answers to a series of specific questions. For the qualitative researcher, each interview is unique, with intense questioning and a less formal structure. Questions might be open, and, depending on the answers from the respondents, new directions might be taken by the researcher, making the process anything but rigid or reproducible.

Qualitative research methodologies have their roots in various academic disciplines and philosophical schools of thought. One of the common and enduring features of qualitative research is that the philosophies underpinning the methodological approach are evident in the design and execution of the study. When reading qualitative research studies it is common to see researchers discuss the philosophical position they have adopted in the preamble to the study or at the very least state who or what has informed their approach. The NMC proficiency 4.1 requires the nurse to 'demonstrate and apply an understanding of what is important to people and how to use this knowledge to ensure their needs for safety, dignity, privacy, comfort and sleep can be met, acting as a role model for others in providing evidence based person-centred care'. This identifies the need for nurses to engage with, at the very least, the methods of qualitative research in their practice so that they might better understand what patients want from their care – as you will do when you undertake Activity 2.1. In order to continue their development as competent professionals, as well as using qualitative methods in their day-to-day work with people, nurses should familiarise themselves with the messages that qualitative research adds to the cumulative knowledge underpinning modern nursing practice.

Platform 6 requires nurses to: 'make a key contribution to the continuous monitoring and quality improvement of care and treatment in order to enhance health outcomes and people's experience of nursing and related care'; also to 'assess risks to safety or experience and take appropriate action to manage those, putting the best interests, needs and preferences of people first'. Nurses should be able to respond to feedback from a wide range of sources in order to 'enhance health outcomes and people's experience of nursing and related care', reflecting the messages learned from qualitative research. The issues that qualitative research often highlight are to do with the quality of the experience of care, so gaining an understanding of qualitative research methodologies links closely to the potential for improving nursing practice.

Concept summary: qualitative research

It is worth thinking for a moment about the philosophy underpinning qualitative research methodologies before exploring the questions they attempt to answer and the methods they employ. Qualitative research asks questions about the nature of reality; it regards reality as being both **subjective** and multiple. This means that qualitative researchers start from the viewpoint that reality is constructed by individuals from their interpretations of what is around them. This construction of reality is subject to personal interpretation and differs from individual to individual. Indeed, the viewpoint of the individual can change over time and in response to life events – for example, becoming chronically ill.

A key characteristic of qualitative research that makes it different from quantitative research is that it does not try to generalise its findings (that is, it does not claim that because this is how one group of people see the world, then all people like them view the world in the same way).

Instead of looking for how the findings of the study might generalise to the wider population, qualitative research often refers to **transferability**. Transferability refers to how much the findings of qualitative research might be able to be applied (transferred) to other settings. This is not really an objective measure of the worth of the research but is seen by many qualitative researchers as something which is down to the interpretation of the person reading the paper (Pope and Mays, 2020; Elo et al., 2014). This is reminiscent of the question from NICE (2015) we cited in Chapter 1 about the applicability of research to people other than those involved in the research. Answering this question in the qualitative sense for nurses reading and considering adopting research is a matter of judgement; therefore, the quality of the write-up of the research paper is important. One way in which the researcher maintains a true reflection of the views and thoughts of the participants in the research is to represent what they have said word for word in the results, so that the meaning, and potential transferability, is not lost in interpretation.

The different qualitative methodologies have evolved to answer different questions. The questions they answer are obviously related in some way to the academic disciplines from which they evolved (Table 2.2). What this means for the qualitative

Methodology	Academic roots
Phenomenology	Philosophy, psychology, sociology
Grounded theory	Sociology (specifically **symbolic interactionism**)
Ethnography	Sociology, cultural anthropology
Case study research	Social sciences

Table 2.2   The academic roots of the qualitative methodologies

researcher is not always clear and, as stated above, not all qualitative enquiry lends itself to being neatly pigeon-holed to one or other methodology. Often qualitative research is called just that – qualitative research – but the approach is normally informed by the assumptions of the paradigm or underpinning philosophy. This failure to identify an exact methodology is, in fact, not a failure at all. Rather, it is a response to the need to be flexible and pragmatic in order to achieve the aims of the study. The overarching philosophy, or, more correctly, **epistemology** (theory of knowledge), remains the same no matter which methodology is adopted (and even if no methodology at all is adopted). The nature of reality, at least for qualitative methods of enquiry, is both individual and varied.

The approach chosen to answer a qualitative question is at least in part dictated by the question itself. As can be seen in Table 2.3, there are specific words associated with different research methodologies. For example, in phenomenology, the focus of which is on an in-depth understanding of a given phenomenon (or experience), the aim of the research is sometimes stated as being to describe the *essence* of a phenomenon (essence in this sense can be thought of as similar to the essence of a flavour used in cooking – for example, vanilla essence, which is the distilled-down and essential flavour of vanilla – you only need a few drops to get the full flavour in a large cake). It is the understanding of the essence, gained through exploring an individual's perceived 'lived experience', that points to, or from which might emerge, a greater understanding of the phenomenon of interest.

A further characteristic of qualitative research is that qualitative researchers try to get close to the person, or people, they are researching. The relationship between

Methodology	Words used in questions
Phenomenology	Describe, experiences, meaning, essence
Grounded theory	Generate, develop, propositions, process, substantive theory
Ethnography	Culture-sharing group, behaviour, language, cultural portrait, cultural themes
Case study research	Single or collective cases, event, process, programme, individual

Table 2.3   Types of words in questions used by different qualitative methodologies
Source: adapted from Creswell and Poth (2017).

the researcher and the researched is part of the research process and is fundamental to obtaining the insider perspective (**emic**) that qualitative research seeks. As well as getting close to the researched, the researcher also explores and expresses their own values about a topic of research before the research starts. This means that anyone reading the published research can form an opinion not only of what the researcher writes about the topic being investigated but also the reasons why the researcher came to these conclusions. The quality of the description of the process and the researcher's position in relation to the subject being studied provides readers with the tools to judge the transferability of the findings of the research to their own area of practice.

Activity 2.2 Reflection

Consider what you think you know about living with a chronic or life-limiting disease. Draw on your experiences to date and the understandings you have gained in your training and practice as a nurse. Now spend some quality time discussing with a family member or friend who has a chronic or life-limiting condition what living with the disease means for them. Compare and contrast the different emphases you both put on elements of the disease, why this might be and what has influenced the distinct positions you both take. Now consider how you can take what you have learnt from this reflection into your working life and how you will transfer this learning. You should also consider how what you have learnt from one discussion might not be enough to inform your understanding of living with disease in general, that is, the limits to transferability.

An outline of what you might find is given at the end of the chapter.

Qualitative research is inductive in its approach to problem solving. 'Inductive' means that the research moves from a specific idea to something more general and theoretical (see Figure 1.2 in Chapter 1). The research question itself is quite broad and open. Inductive researchers do not set out with an idea of what they might find, as one does with a hypothesis, for example (see Figure 1.1 in Chapter 1, and Chapter 4). Instead they allow the data they collect to lead them towards an understanding of the phenomenon under investigation. In grounded theory, for example, this inductive reasoning leads researchers to the point where they create a new theory for understanding the social process under investigation.

Concept summary: inductive reasoning

If you are struggling with the concept of inductive reasoning, think about the methods employed by detectives in popular detective novels and television programmes

(Continued)

(Continued)

(for example, Inspector Barnaby or Endeavour). These fictional detectives collect clues surrounding a given case and use these to construct hypotheses. At this stage they are acting inductively – they allow the information to lead them instead of looking for clues to support any preconceived notion about what might have happened. Once a number of clues have been gathered, the data are analysed and a hypothesis is formed; the detective then becomes more deductive, looking for clues and seeking out information that will support the hypothesis he or she has formed. This example not only demonstrates the differences between inductive and deductive approaches to research, it also demonstrates that the two can be used usefully together to help gain a full understanding of an individual or an occurrence.

Activity 2.3   Reflection

Life events are things that have happened to you or to others within your lifetime that affect your attitudes and opinions. Significant life events may include becoming a parent, experiencing illness or trauma or the death of a loved one. Other life events are experienced by people collectively and may include natural disasters or terrorist activities that change the way in which we see the world for ever.

What life events have you experienced which have changed your view of things? Why?

An outline of what you might find is given at the end of the chapter.

Weaknesses of qualitative research

The very nature of qualitative research lays it open to many criticisms. The subjective nature of qualitative enquiry means that it is hard to replicate – that is, people's opinions and attitudes, beliefs and ideals are different from place to place and from time to time. So the opinions, attitudes, ideals and beliefs that are common in one setting are not necessarily the same in another because they are affected by characteristics such as nationality, culture and life experiences. Furthermore, subjectivity is so intertwined with context that a single event can change a person's perspective forever as the context of that individual's life changes; think about your answer to Activities 2.2 and 2.3, for example, and how your experience of the COVID-19 pandemic has affected your view of life. This means that the findings of a qualitative study are inextricably linked to the people who were studied, the time in which they were studied and the prevalent cultural and social norms.

The fact that the findings of qualitative research are so subjective and so bound to the context in which the research is undertaken means the findings are hard to generalise. In turn, this means that it may be hard to justify applying the findings of any qualitative enquiry away from the setting in which the study was undertaken. That said, qualitative researchers claim, and rightly so, that the purpose of their enquiry is not necessarily to create findings that are statistically generalisable but to create what Popay et al. (1998) call *logical generalisations*, which relate to similar situations or occurrences. This means the applicability of the findings of a qualitative study to a similar setting, or phenomenon, is not a matter of scientific certainty, but, as Polit and Beck (2020) identify, such transferability relies on whether the researchers have provided a rich enough description of the sample and the study context for the reader to be able to make this judgement for themselves.

Qualitative research has also been criticised for lacking scientific **rigour** and **credibility** because the processes involved are subject to the values and beliefs of the person undertaking the research. Qualitative researchers counter this by saying that they recognise, and in some cases even welcome, the subjectivity of the qualitative research process. The fact that they acknowledge that their presence and actions within the research setting may affect the outcomes means that everyone is aware of the issue anyway, and that the results of the study can be read in this context. Or as Pope and Mays (2020) state, qualitative researchers:

> *should make their personal and intellectual biases plain at the outset of any research reports to enhance the credibility of their findings and help the reader interpret the findings and conclusions.*

Where qualitative research is concerned, the importance of writing up the process and findings of the research in full cannot be overemphasised. It is the completeness of the write-up which enables nurses to decide whether and how they should apply the findings of the research to their own practice.

Phenomenology

Phenomenology has a short, colourful and eclectic history. Phenomenology has variously been applied to the study of people, ethics, law, aesthetics and architecture (Moran, 2000). There are a number of distinct philosophical tendencies within phenomenology, but at their heart lies the definition of phenomenology as a research methodology which is concerned with understanding an experience from the **first-person perspective** (Zahavi, 2018).

It is this requisite of accessing the nature of the 'first-person' experience that lies at the heart of phenomenology, which establishes its strong emic credentials. In health and social care, phenomenology is widely used to aid understanding of phenomena such as the lived experience of neuropathic pain following spinal cord injury (Heath Hearn et al., 2017), the lived experience and understanding of psychosis (Brew et al., 2017) and the individual and shared identities of women with Down's syndrome (Groves et al., 2017).

Key features

Edmund Husserl is credited as being the founder of modern phenomenology; his method of studying human consciousness and experience is characterised by an approach that is often termed **descriptive phenomenology**. Husserl's approach relied heavily on the fact that humans are by nature reflective beings who make sense of their world using the evidence available to them via their physical senses. The purpose of descriptive phenomenology is to access the essence of an object or an experience as the individual experiencing it sees it – no more and no less – what Crotty (1998) famously describes as the *ultimate structure of consciousness*. While accessing this experience through the research subject (usually via interview), researchers put out of their minds any preconceived ideas they have about the object or experience, a process known as **epoching** or **bracketing** (Zahavi, 2018).

Of course, in reality it is virtually impossible to put to one side one's feelings or prior knowledge of an event or an experience, and most phenomenological researchers describe their own preconceptions about an issue being researched prior to starting the data collection – that is, they are reflexive. This 'laying bare', as it is called, allows individuals reading the research to judge for themselves whether the preconceived ideas of the researcher have had an impact on that person's interpretation of what the research subjects have said.

Concept summary: epoching or bracketing

Epoching or bracketing is the process by which researchers put to one side all of their preconceptions and ideas about the topic they are studying. By putting aside all preconceived ideas about the world or the phenomenon being studied, the researcher can allow the inductive process of coming to an understanding of things through the use of the data as they emerge to take place.

Martin Heidegger, a student of Husserl's, modified the descriptive phenomenological approach. His **interpretative phenomenology** is refined by his attention to the **hermeneutics**, or analysis/interpretation, of human experience. Unlike Husserl's approach, Heidegger's view is that human existence, and experience, is made up of our interpretations of what we see, feel and experience (Parahoo, 2014). Hence, Heidegger's hermeneutical phenomenology relies heavily on accessing people's expressed perspective on their lived experience, which is intertwined with and influenced by their social context. Heidegger believed our understanding comes from entering the world of another person and discovering the understandings and wisdom found there (Polit and Beck, 2020).

More recently, **interpretative phenomenological analysis** has attempted to work with the interpretative nature of phenomenological enquiry. The emphasis remains on accessing the participants' perception of the phenomenon, but it further recognises that this is itself an interpretation of the lived world and that researchers themselves will apply an interpretation to the research subjects' interpretation (Smith, 2016). That is, the researcher will try to make sense of the subjects' attempts to make sense of their world.

Streubert and Carpenter (2010) helpfully identify three questions that the researcher should ask before setting out to undertake a phenomenological study:

1. Is there a need for more clarity of understanding of the phenomenon?
2. Will the experiences of the subjects provide this information?
3. Have I got the time, resources, skills and personality necessary to undertake this study?

The first and second questions help in deciding if the approach is the right one; they eliminate doubt about the need for and the approach to answering the question posed. The third question is more practical and could apply equally well to any research enquiry (as discussed at the end of Chapter 1). The nature of phenomenology, however, is such that it requires researchers to engage with the process in a great deal of depth, over an extended period of time, while recognising their own biases and subjective opinions.

Sampling in phenomenological research

The sampling method used in phenomenological research has, by definition, to be a **purposive** one. Purposive samples select people who have experienced the phenomenon of interest. So, for example, if we wanted to know what it was like to have multiple sclerosis, then we would approach and research people who have the disease. The sample selection will be determined by the exact question we are seeking to answer. So, again, if we were interested in what it was like to be a mother living with multiple sclerosis, then we would approach only mothers who were living with the disease.

In common with all qualitative methodologies, phenomenology seeks to gain in-depth understanding of a topic that is credible and might extrapolate to similar situations. Generalisability (the ability to generalise the findings of a study beyond the sample researched) is not as important in qualitative research (see the discussion on generalisability in Chapter 1) as it is in quantitative research, and therefore, as in all qualitative methodologies, the sample sizes used are quite small. Various sources suggest that a sample of between three and ten individuals is sufficient for the purposes of this kind of study (Creswell and Creswell, 2018). In reality, the sample size may be determined by time, money and availability of study subjects. As with many qualitative studies, a **convenience sample** is often used. Also in common with other qualitative study samples, because of the in-depth nature of this type of study the small sample can provide data that are both rich and deep, reflecting the intended purpose of qualitative methodologies.

The ideal way to determine the size of the sample to be studied in phenomenological research is to analyse the data from the interviews as the study progresses, stopping the interview process when no new themes are emerging from the data. The point at which there appear to be no new ideas emerging from the interviews is often referred to as **data saturation**.

Concept summary: data saturation

Data saturation is a term used in many qualitative methodologies to define the point at which there appears to be no further benefit to be gained from continuing to collect data about a topic of interest. The use of data saturation as identifying the point at which data collection stops is as much practical as academic. This is because qualitative methodologies (unlike quantitative methodologies) cannot use statistical sample size calculations as a point at which to stop the collection of data for a study because they are not concerned with collecting numerate data.

Methods used in data collection

Data for phenomenological research are invariably collected using interviews. The reason for this is that interviews allow the researcher to explore in depth an issue with an individual by adjusting questioning according to what the respondent is saying, probing the meaning behind the responses given and thereby gaining insight into the experience of the individual (Brinkmann and Kvale, 2014).

Case study

In their phenomenological study of access to mental health services in rural settings, Jensen et al. (2020) interviewed eight mental health professionals. They found that the professionals believed there to be distinct cultures in rural areas, rural working mental health professionals face unique challenges, there are barriers to accessing mental health support in rural locations and mental health professionals needed to be innovative in order to overcome the barriers.

Phenomenological studies often use either **unstructured** or **semi-structured interview** methodologies (as opposed to the more rigid structured interview that might be undertaken as part of market research). More flexible interviewing structures allow

41

the interviewer to explore the issues that are of importance to the interviewee. This exploratory interview method fits better with the aims of phenomenological research, which are to explore the meaning or essence of an experience (such as the experience of providing mental health services) for the individual. Open questions are used (also called open-ended questions), as these allow participants to take the discussion in the direction which is important to them rather than the interview following a path set by the interviewer.

Interviews conducted in this manner often use topic, or interview, guides rather than interview schedules; topic guides both keep interviewers focused on the questions they need to ask but also allow them to respond flexibly to the answers the interviewee gives. Where there is limited knowledge on a topic prior to undertaking the interviews, some researchers use focus group work to gain the necessary insight (Pederson et al., 2016).

Some researchers have used focus groups as a means of collecting data for phenomenological studies. While these are quicker than a series of one-to-one interviews, the disadvantage is that they collect a group consensus view and may not always gain insight into the actual feelings or interpretations of the individuals present. These difficulties may be more acute when the topic being researched is in a sensitive area. This approach also risks not getting to the essence of the experience as a consensus view rarely allows this to happen.

Grounded theory

Grounded theory is a qualitative methodology used to analyse social processes. It can be thought of as a methodology that tries to generate new, or explore and expand upon existing, ideas or *theories* about a human activity by examining people's perceptions and understandings of it. Once the theory is derived, its application to a social interaction can be viewed as providing a potential explanation of the important social processes that have been derived (grounded) from the data collected, hence 'grounded theory'.

Grounded theory research is used to generate theories about practice and understanding from many different areas of healthcare, including: the processes which go into enabling patients in the general practice setting (Desborough et al., 2016); understanding the experiences and preferences of palliative care patients (Sinclair et al., 2016); and understanding nurses' approaches to delivering spiritual care (Ramezani et al., 2017).

Key features

Of the qualitative approaches to research, grounded theory is the most systematic in its approach. Philosophically and academically it is closely linked to sociology – the study of people in society and social groups. Grounded theory is one of the most popular qualitative methodologies used by nurse researchers.

The whole grounded theory approach to enquiry is based on the notion that a social group, or groups, has shared social interpretations that are not always well described (Glaser and Strauss, 1967). Barney Glaser and Anselm Strauss, the founders of modern grounded theory, expressly criticised sociology because, at the time, sociologists were seeking evidence to support existing theories rather than using evidence to create new theory (being deductive rather than inductive). Glaser and Strauss's argument, quite reasonably, suggested that if sociology was to accept that a theory had any basis in truth, then the data for the generation of the theory, which in social and natural science means something more than a hunch or speculation, had to precede the creation of the theory and not the other way round! Grounded theory systematically applies procedural steps to explore social phenomena and derive a theory that explains people's understanding of those phenomena. Strauss and Corbin (1990, p23) explain a grounded theory as:

> one that is inductively derived from the study of the phenomenon it represents. That is, it is discovered, developed, and provisionally verified through systematic data collection and analysis of data pertaining to that phenomenon. Therefore, data collection, analysis, and theory stand in reciprocal relationship with each other. One does not begin with a theory, then prove it. Rather, one begins with an area of study and what is relevant to that area is allowed to emerge.

The aim of grounded theory is, therefore, the discovery of theoretical explanations for, and about, a particular phenomenon.

Like all qualitative research, then, grounded theory focuses on meanings coming from the phenomena being studied, rather than on forming a hypothesis or theory before starting the study. Grounded theory, however, is regarded more as a theory-building strategy in social science research whereas ethnography, as we shall see, is more descriptive. The requirement on the grounded theorist is to remain sensitive and adhere to the methodology at all times (Reay et al., 2016). Grounded theorists record their observations of phenomena of interest before systematically testing their understanding by looking for evidence to support, or refute, the theory being built.

Concept summary: theories and hypotheses

At this point it is worth thinking about the nature of a theory and a hypothesis. The word hypothesis can be thought of as a combination of the two words *hypo* (below) and *thesis* (well-developed idea), while a theory may be regarded as a hypothesis that is supported by the collection of evidence such that it is closer to being established fact. It is important when thinking about the nature of qualitative enquiry using grounded theory methodology that the ultimate aim is to generate a theory, that is, an idea or concept supported by empirical facts.

Sampling in grounded theory research

A **homogeneous** sample of people who have all shared the same experience, or gone through the same process, is the starting point for sampling in grounded theory research. The sample is, therefore, purposive (selected for the purpose of the study). The sample needs to be broad enough to enable the researcher to draw on the experiences of enough people to come to some conclusions about the commonalities of the experience. Often a convenience sample will be used, which consists of people who are identified because they attend a particular hospital clinic, social group or a university course.

After interviewing the initial sample the grounded theorist will analyse the interviews for the data that emerge and start to create initial theories about the phenomenon of interest (for more about this process in grounded theory, see Chapter 3). This initial and ongoing analysis of data will lead researchers to ask further questions around the area of interest and may lead to them recruiting further subjects to the study in order to help answer emerging questions or to consolidate an emerging theory further. This process is called **theoretical sampling**.

Concept summary: theoretical sampling

Theoretical sampling is a sampling method that is usually confined to grounded theory research. Theoretical sampling occurs as researchers build new theories and ideas from the data they have collected; they test these new theories by interviewing more subjects, who are purposively selected, to see if the new theories still hold true. Theoretical sampling is also known as 'handy' sampling.

Methods used in data collection

Grounded theorists collect data from a variety of sources, including case studies, interviews, documentary evidence and participant observation. Interviews remain the most widely used mechanism of data collection because it is only during interview that the researcher can get to the heart of the individual's interpretation of a phenomenon. In order to get to such meaning, the interviews are usually indepth and unstructured or semi-structured to allow the interviewer to respond to the ideas and statements coming from the participant rather than boxing the interviewee in by the use of questions that may be irrelevant to them (Brinkmann and Kvale, 2014).

Case study

In a study by Eslami Akbar et al. (2017), 15 clinical nurses were purposively and theoretically sampled to undergo unstructured interviews with field notes. The theory generated suggested that nurses cope with job stress through making an effort to cope with individual situations, that nurses recognised the impact of their personal abilities to cope as well as the impact of their environment. They also noted how they made a 'comprehensive effort' to stay calm even in stressful situations.

Grounded theory research methods are well structured and well developed, and it is hard to separate the process of data collection from the process of data analysis since what one finds determines how long one continues to collect data. Data collection and analysis take place simultaneously and, as can be seen in the example, often includes **field notes**. This process informs the sampling that continues until no new data to inform the emergent (grounded) theory are forthcoming. In common with all qualitative methodologies, Engward and Davis (2015) state that grounded theorists must be reflexive, that is, open and honest about their preconceptions and ideas coming into the study, so that the reader can draw a complete picture of how they have come to the conclusions they have.

Concept summary: field notes

Field notes are the notes a researcher takes when out in the 'field', that is, collecting data. These notes prompt them to issues such as body language, facial expression, tone of voice and other cues which may be forgotten at a later date when analysing the core data such as interview transcripts.

Ethnography

Ethnographic research seeks to describe and interpret activity within social groups. It seeks to understand the culture within a group, where culture is defined as the behaviours, norms and meaning of the group from the viewpoint of an insider, that is, a member of the group (the emic perspective). Ethnography has its roots in **anthropology**, which means the study of humans and is taken from the Greek *anthropos* (human) and *logia* (study). Ethnography is used to study all manner of social relationships and realities – for example: whether nurse-led units are really nurse-led (Farrell et al., 2017); introducing nurse practitioners into an interprofessional team (Kvarnstrom et al., 2017); and the use of non-pharmacological interventions in managing patients with dementia in the care home setting (Blackhouse et al., 2016).

Concept summary: emic perspective

An emic perspective is the insider's view. In ethnography this would be the view of the culture from a member of the group being studied. This is the opposite of the **etic** perspective, which is the view of someone else *looking in* at the same culture – in this case, perhaps, the ethnographer. If you are struggling with the concepts of emic and etic, think about how different people view living with disease, which we explored in Activity 2.2.

Key features

The key feature of ethnography as a qualitative research methodology is that it involves long-term study of a group by the researcher, who becomes both an observer and a participant in the group – this is often termed **participant observation**. Because the researchers are very much part of the group being studied, they will influence how the group behaves – and how the group behaves may influence them. The observation is not neutral, hence the use of the term *participant*.

Pope and Mays (2020) note one of the potential pitfalls facing the ethnographic researcher is that of *going native*. What this means is that some ethnographers become immersed in the culture they are studying and start not only to behave like the group being studied but build emotional and social allegiances and feel like one of the group. Depending on your viewpoint, this 'going native' can be seen as either a problem or a benefit to the research process.

Case study

James Patrick, who studied gang culture in Glasgow in the 1950s, left Glasgow in a hurry after only 12 sessions with the gang from the Maryhill district of the city. Patrick had found the level of violence unacceptable and was unable to study the gang any longer. He did, however, manage to publish his study of the gang's culture after a suitable period of time, which served to protect the gang members' identities (Patrick, 1973).

Sampling in ethnographic research

Access to a group for study may involve the researcher in seeking the help of a **gate-keeper**. In this sense, a gatekeeper is someone already in a group who will not only allow the researcher access to the group but also introduce that person to group members and even help the researcher to integrate into the group. Classically, researchers have downplayed their own role in a group in an attempt to maintain some level of objectivity, or artificial distance, and credibility. However, it is now more common for researchers to explore their own part in the group as part of the research – in a sense creating their own autobiography of belonging to the group. We have discussed the importance of researchers describing the research process in some detail in order to inform readers' decision making about the applicability of the research to their own workplace – this is of special importance for ethnographic research.

Some ethnographers use their place of work as a rich source of data for ethnography, seeking to derive meaning from the interactions that take place there. In this context, the ability and opportunities for data collection are vast and the insights gained may be great. There are some issues with this approach, however, as one may start off 'native' and therefore lack objectivity – and there remain ethical questions about the informed consent of colleagues who may forget that they are now a subject of study as well as being colleagues in the classic sense. Researching in one's place of work, however, is a rich source of information and understanding. Therefore, as long as in the write-up the researcher lays bare the influences on the way he or she has formed opinions and understandings of the data collected, then it remains a legitimate place of study.

Case study

In their **ethnographic study** of surgical team communications and relationships, Tørring et al. (2019) observed and interviewed members of 39 surgical teams over a 10-month period. The observer only observed and did not participate (passive observing). Tørring also kept field notes relating to their observations. This study identified four different communication and relationship patterns among the surgical teams: proactive and intuitive communication, silent and ordinary communication, inattentive and ambiguous communication, and contradictory and highly dynamic communication.

Methods used in data collection

Creswell and Creswell (2018) identify how data collection in ethnography which is focused on the culture of a group includes examining artifacts (things of value to the group), interviews, observations and a number of case studies (detailed reviews). The data collection approaches used by ethnographers are therefore many and varied.

Activity 2.4   Critical thinking

Given that ethnographers are often studying groups about which they have little knowledge, and with whom they have few connections, what problems might they encounter when trying to collect data for their study? How might they overcome some of these problems? Do you think it is possible to remain entirely objective at the same time as immersing oneself in the activities of the group being studied?

There is a possible answer at the end of the chapter.

Participant observation is the key, but not the only, method used in data collection. Being part of a group allows the researcher to gain a perspective on the norms of the group, its use of language and its shared values. The ethnographer keeps copious notes of the interactions within the group and between him/herself and members of the group, often reflecting on and deciphering meaning from casual conversations and interactions. Gathering and reflecting on information requires a level of practised detachment on the part of the researcher that allows that person to see meaning within normal everyday interactions. In the study by Tørring et al. (2019), the research fails to mention any discussion of, or reflection on, the researcher's observations with another member of the research team to try to maintain some objectivity, which would be realistic to expect.

It would be reasonable to ask: what is the purpose of prolonged observation? Surely any insights can be gained during interviews or focus group discussions? Verbal data collection methods have a significant role to play in the understanding of the group. There are, however, things of which groups may share a common knowledge or understanding that they may not think important and would therefore not raise during interview. Such things, often termed **tacit knowledge**, may not come up in conversation but will emerge from the interactions of the group. One of the important roles of ethnography is to discover, and describe, this sort of important hidden detail. What people say they do and what they say they hold important may or may not reflect how they behave; in that respect gaining a complete picture of a group requires collection of data gained through both observation and interview. One of the strengths of the study by Tørring et al. (2019) was that it took place over a long period of time and one might therefore expect a realistic view of staff behaviours to be observed.

Concept summary: tacit knowledge

Tacit knowledge is a common feature of nursing (and, indeed, many professions). There are understandings that we gain about human interaction and the delivery of care that we

(Continued)

(Continued)

know, but just don't know why we know them. Not only do we forget why we may know something, but we also sometimes forget where we learnt it. As such, this knowledge is then just part of our body of knowledge as nurses – something that does not usually need to be discussed within our professional body but that is unknown to others outside nursing. It might be described as knowing as a result of informal social learning. A word of caution, however: tacit knowledge could be inaccurate if the initial set of actions is wrong and this learning goes unchallenged – for example where new knowledge is not subjected to critical reflection.

Other data collected in ethnographic research may include pictures, symbols and images that have meaning to the members of the group and that allow the researcher to convey these meanings to the people reading the research. Such symbols may give clues to the shared understandings and identity of the group and promote deeper understanding.

More structured data collection is a common feature of ethnographic studies, which often means undertaking interviews. Because of the long-term relationships developed during the course of a study, interviews may actually occur during everyday conversations and interactions – the content of which are captured in field notes. Many ethnographers use in-depth formal interviews during the course of their data collection, employing **open questions** designed to allow respondents to answer in whatever way they feel is correct without leading them towards an answer.

It is easy to imagine from this description that data collection proceeds in a well-defined and planned manner; however, this certainly is not always the case. Indeed, the three key activities of data collection described above happen simultaneously and cyclically. As such, data collection in ethnography can be quite messy and challenging, and requires detailed note-taking, constant reflection, and development and amendment of methods depending on what is found, when and how. It is both inductive and iterative.

Case study/biographic research

Creswell and Poth (2017, p97) define case study research as: *an exploration of a 'bounded system' or a case (or multiple cases) over time through detailed, in-depth data collection involving multiple sources of information (e.g. observations, interviews, audio-visual material, and documents and reports).* While this definition is correct, it may appear to be misleading since Creswell and Poth are using the term 'bounded system' to refer to any of the following: an individual, a collection of individuals, a system, an organisation or an intervention.

Case study research is the least well-understood approach to qualitative enquiry. It is a widely held view among the research community that case study research is not useful as an insight into a wider group or other systems and its usefulness is restricted to the early stage of qualitative enquiry in hypothesis generation to be evaluated by subsequent larger-scale investigations. This view is increasingly being challenged as more literature emerges providing structure to case studies as a methodology (Hancock and Algozzine, 2017). Bailey et al. (2016) used a critical incident case study approach to understanding the experiences of patients with advanced chronic obstructive pulmonary disease; Jangland et al. (2016) employed a multi-stage qualitative case study approach to understand the care experiences of patients with acute abdominal pain; while Ansar et al. (2017) used a case study approach to understand the challenges in accessing healthcare for involuntary migrants.

Key features

According to Yin (2018) and Hancock and Algozzine (2017), a case study approach to qualitative questioning might be considered when: the point of the study is answering 'how' and 'why' questions; it is not possible to manipulate the behaviour of the individuals involved in the study; the boundaries between the phenomenon and context are unclear; and it is desirable to study the contextual conditions because it is believed that they are of **relevance** to the phenomenon being studied. Approaches to case study research are quite flexible and not bounded by philosophical underpinnings in the way methodologies like phenomenology are. It is because it is viewed as being a highly flexible qualitative methodology that case study research is increasingly popular among researchers (Hyett et al., 2014).

Sampling in case study research

In common with most qualitative methods, the starting point for the sample for the research is individuals who constitute the system being researched or have experience of the intervention of interest; that is, the sampling method is purposive. Some research commentators, Creswell and Poth (2017) among them, consider that sampling unusual cases (those whose experience of the topic under discussion is not the norm) is useful in some collective case studies as they provide a broader perspective on the issue. What is clear in case study research is that a lot of thought needs to go into what exactly one is studying because there is a world of difference between studying an individual and studying a process or organisation.

Methods used in data collection

A feature of case study research is the use of multiple sources of data. Potential sources of data include documentation, interviews, archived records, objects, observation and pictures. Unlike other qualitative research methodologies, case study researchers can use quantitative data in order to gain a fuller insight into a phenomenon being studied. Data from the many diverse sources are then joined together in the analysis, like putting together the pieces of a puzzle.

Bringing the pieces of the puzzle together like this allows the researcher to gain a more holistic view of the individual or system being studied. Bringing together data from many diverse sources adds strength to the findings as the various strands of enquiry are woven together to improve upon the understanding of the phenomenon under study.

Of course, there is always the potential pitfall with this type of eclectic approach that too much data will be collected and that it will prove overwhelming to process all the data in a meaningful manner. To this end there are many advantages of using a computerised database for case study research.

Case study

In their qualitative case study about the enablers for creating an interprofessional team response to COVID-19 in a critical care environment, Hales et al. (2020) collected data from a purposive sample of individuals using field notes, email correspondence and email and verbal feedback. They discovered the response to the pandemic and successful creation of emergency care teams was a function of working in well-supported interprofessional teams.

Chapter summary

In this chapter we have seen how qualitative research employs inductive methods in order to describe and understand the diverse ways in which people behave and experience and understand the world.

We have identified the major methodologies used within qualitative research in healthcare and have discovered they all use methods which allow them to see the world from the point of view of the person(s) being studied. We have seen that qualitative research is used to answer a number of different questions, and certain methodologies and methods are best suited to specific types of question. The ways in which samples are chosen – and the reasons for these – have been identified, as have the key methods used to collect data in qualitative research.

We have seen that qualitative research is important to nursing in extending our understanding of how people experience the care that we deliver. If we review the key messages of qualitative research, it is straightforward to see how an understanding of the approaches to and tools used in qualitative research add an extra dimension to our ability as nurses to deliver high-quality care.

Activities: brief outline answers

Activity 2.2   Reflection (page 36)

What you consider to be important elements of disease and what someone living with disease considers to be important may or may not be the same. As a care professional you might identify some health-related aspects of the disease as being of paramount importance, while the person you talked to may have different perspectives on what is important, e.g. they may consider their social care needs, or the need to look after their cat, as of paramount importance.

It is likely there is some overlap in your understanding, since as humans we share commonality of experience, but the importance placed on different elements will doubtless vary from person to person and in the same person according to experience. For us, as nurses, this points squarely to the need to keep the patient firmly at the centre of what we do and how we do it, since it is patients' meaning which is important and not ours.

Activity 2.3   Reflection (page 37)

Life experiences have an effect on the person that we become. While nurses are often encouraged to be empathetic towards their patients it is hard to become so without some life experiences to draw on. Experiencing life-changing events such as pain, embarrassment or bereavement allows us to understand better what some of our patients experience while in our care.

Activity 2.4   Critical thinking (page 48)

Getting into and understanding the values of a group requires the ethnographer to establish a rapport with a member of the group of interest (a gatekeeper). This group member then becomes the means to gain access to the group and may help the researcher to identify the shared values and common understandings of the group. This is not always easy as many groups have a language of their own and share a collective understanding of issues, symbols and ideas not immediately obvious to an outsider. Think about the language you are used to in the practice setting and how hard it was to sit through a handover when you were new to nursing. The key to success is, therefore, time and communication with a key informant within the group who can give meaning to new ideas, processes and concepts in much the same way as a clinical mentor does for the student nurse. The ability to remain objective during data collection for an ethnographic study will be affected by the amount of time and the intensity of the new experience. For the novice researcher this may be achieved by using a research supervisor or a research buddy who can provide a sounding board and a reality check when needed.

Further reading

Creswell, JW and Poth, CN (2017) *Qualitative Inquiry and Research Design: Choosing among Five Approaches* (4th edn). Thousand Oaks: Sage.

A great text for understanding the differences between the qualitative research methodologies.

Parahoo, K (2014) *Nursing Research: Principles, Process and Issues* (3rd edn). London: Palgrave Macmillan.

Chapter 4 is a very useful introduction to the principles of qualitative research.

Streubert, HJ and Carpenter, DR (2010) *Qualitative Research in Nursing: Advancing the Humanistic Imperative* (5th edn). London: Lippincott Williams & Wilkins.

Chapters 1 and 2 provide a very accessible introduction to the philosophy and conduct of qualitative research.

Zahavi, D (2018) *Phenomenology: The Basics*. London: Routledge.

A really accessible introduction to phenomenology.

Useful websites

www.analytictech.com/mb870/introtoGT.htm An introduction to grounded theory.

www.qualres.org A comprehensive website covering all aspects of qualitative research.

www.phenomenologyonline.com An easy-to-use and understand resource for people exploring phenomenological methodologies.

https://tqr.nova.edu/websites A site pointing to lots of qualitative web resources.

sru.soc.surrey.ac.uk/index.html *Social Research Update* is published quarterly by the Department of Sociology, University of Surrey.

www.ncrm.ac.uk/resources/index.php The resource page of the National Centre for Research Methods – look especially at the qualitative research video podcasts.

Chapter 3 Data collection methods and analysis in qualitative research

Chapter aims

After reading this chapter, you will be able to:

- identify the major data collection methods used in qualitative research;
- describe the advantages and disadvantages of the data collection methods used in qualitative research;
- describe the key elements of data analysis in qualitative research;
- demonstrate awareness of the quality issues related to data management in qualitative research.

Introduction

In the previous chapter qualitative research methodologies were identified as a means of answering questions about people's opinions, attitudes, feelings and interpretation of experience. This chapter identifies the appropriate data collection methods (research tools) within qualitative research and explains how they meet the aims of the chosen methodology. It explores how the data are collected, and the pros and cons of the verbal and observational data collection methods used within the qualitative methodologies.

The aim of this chapter is to introduce the reader to the general principles of the approaches and some of their strengths and weaknesses rather than to provide an exhaustive exploration of the methods used in qualitative research. Readers are advised to access the further reading suggested at the end of the chapter if they want further information or guidance on qualitative research methods.

This chapter also looks at data presentation and data analysis in qualitative research and what they serve to demonstrate. It also illuminates some of the ways in which the process of data analysis in the qualitative methodologies can be demonstrated to be rigorous and credible, that is to say, how the quality of the data collection is demonstrated.

Key features

Qualitative methodologies are concerned with people, their actions and the meaning people attach to the activities in which they engage. Capturing people's behaviour and the meanings they attach to it is not something that can be undertaken lightly or superficially. For this reason qualitative researchers often argue that the work that they do is both **deep** and **rich**.

This depth and richness, sometimes referred to as being **thick** (Streubert and Carpenter, 2010), comes from the ability of the methodologies and their associated methods to tap into the meaning of human interaction and of being. These notions are not readily measurable in an empirical sense, nor can they be identified by casual observation or interaction. The data are deep because the research probes answers to move towards a more robust understanding of a topic, and rich because the data captured are full of meaning.

Clearly, any attempt to understand human interaction – or people's understanding of, or feelings about, a topic – requires engagement with the individuals in question. This allows the researcher to gain an insight into the world of the research participants and the meaning they attach to the things that happen there. Engaging with, and understanding, people takes time, effort and perseverance.

As nurses, we are familiar and comfortable with the day-to-day communications and interactions that take place between us and our patients. We undertake clinical observations and gather data to inform our care. The interaction required for qualitative data collection is somewhat deeper than that required in the general nursing setting. Such interactions require not only observation and our interpretation of the observation, but also probing and understanding of the topic from the point of view of the subject of the research – and that is the focus of qualitative research: gaining a view of the understanding of another person, the *emic* perspective.

Concept summary: signs and symptoms

To think about the difference between your understanding of the world and someone else's, think about the difference between signs and symptoms of illness. Signs are things that we can measure and see in other people, for instance, their temperature, pulse and blood pressure. Symptoms must be explained to us by the person experiencing them – for example, pain or anxiety. So, to gain an insight into someone else's world, we need to ask them how they see things, what their experience is and how they interpret it. We cannot gain this just by looking at them, in the same way that we cannot see the symptoms of their illness!

The collection of data within the qualitative methods therefore requires in-depth engagement on the part of the researcher. The researcher is seen as a 'tool of data collection' rather than as someone who uses tools to collect data (as one might use a thermometer when taking a temperature or a sphygmomanometer for recording blood pressure, for example). This is seen as both a key strength and a key weakness of data collection in qualitative research.

The main strength lies in the depth of the data that can be collected. The main weakness is that it is hard either to prevent or detect bias in the data collection. The quality of the processes by which bias is controlled in qualitative data collection and analysis is referred to as its rigour (Cypress, 2017).

One of the key tools for demonstrating the credibility of the qualitative research process is **reflexivity**. Reflexive researchers will identify their own biases and preconceptions through reflection and will present these in the write-up of the research paper. So, unlike the quantitative researcher who tries hard to eliminate bias, the qualitative researcher lives with bias and manages it by presenting it honestly to the reader.

Concept summary: rigour

Rigour refers to the strict processes attached to both data collection and analysis within qualitative research that establishes the credibility and the **dependability** of the findings. The consistency and quality of the data collection processes, the manner in which these are recorded and described, and the quality of the data analysis, as well as its transparency, all add to the rigour that a study can be said to have. A good study will demonstrate that it has been thoroughly rigorous; a poor study will leave questions about the level of rigour used.

The next section explores verbal data collection methods, that is, interviews and focus groups. After that, observation – primarily participant observation – as a tool of qualitative data is discussed.

Interviews

There are a number of ways in which interviews can be undertaken in qualitative research. The choice of interview method, number of interviews and place of interview will depend on the nature of the issue being examined, the methodology being used, the availability of research subjects and the experience of the researcher. It would be misleading to state that a particular style of interviewing belongs to a specific qualitative methodology, as there is limited agreement on this issue even among experienced researchers – although, as we will see, the questions posed by some qualitative methodologies do tend to suggest that one approach to interviewing is used in preference to another. In order to establish credibility and demonstrate rigour, the best research lays out the reasons for the choice of approach to interviewing and how this applies to the topic under investigation.

Interviewing for qualitative research is a skill that requires acquisition and development and improves with practice. Before undertaking an interview there are a number of questions the interviewer needs to ask and answer. Not least among these is, 'What is the purpose of the interview?' This may seem a simplistic question at first glance, but it is one with clear links to the question posed in the study and the choice of research methodology.

In one form of phenomenological research, for example, the interviewer will be seeking to gain a deep insight into the *essence* of the experience being investigated. The nature of the enquiry and the in-depth understanding required would tend to suggest that the interview (or interviews) needs to be lengthy and probing. By contrast, the conversations and data collection the ethnographer undertakes may range from informal or casual conversations to more structured and probing in-depth interviews, depending on the original question.

Despite specific methods apparently belonging to specific methodologies, different researchers will choose to use different data collection methods to answer their research questions even when apparently working within the same methodology. We have already seen that in-depth interviews are widely used in phenomenological research; however, Bradbury-Jones et al. (2009) argue that the use of focus groups in phenomenological research can be beneficial as it opens the participants up to alternative views while stimulating discussion about the topic of interest (see discussion of focus groups later in the chapter). Being subjected to other views and opinions can, they claim, improve understanding and hence refine the views of the participants, leading to higher-quality data collection. Conversely, it may be argued that this potential changing of the opinions and understanding of the participants is contrary to the purpose of phenomenological study, which is to see the world as the research participant sees it. Again neither approach is more wrong or more right, but researchers need to establish their reasons for choosing the method used in order to demonstrate rigour.

Interviews are appropriate when the research question seeks to discover the thoughts, feelings or perceptions of individuals about an issue or experience. They can be used to give context to other data collected during a study by adding an element of interpretation to something observed, for example, in an ethnographic enquiry. They are also beneficial when the topic being investigated is one that may cause embarrassment or that people are likely to be reserved about discussing in a group (e.g. focus group) setting (Tod, 2015).

Activity 3.1 Reflection

Think about how easy it is to discuss sensitive issues in the open ward. How do you make it easier for patients to tell you private and intimate details in the practice setting? What barriers exist to gaining a full and frank insight into the thoughts and feelings of the patients where you work?

There are some possible answers at the end of the chapter.

The standard of NMC proficiency 4.1 highlights the role of the nurse in ensuring the privacy and dignity of people at all times; this is equally valid in the research setting as it is in practice.

Key features

Interviewing as a data collection method requires prior planning. By the time the researcher has reached the point of planning the interview, s/he should already have identified the purpose of the interview and the sample characteristics needed, and have some rough idea of the sample size.

Planning the interview requires the researcher to be clear about what information is wanted and from whom. This relates back strongly to the purpose of the study and the study question, which should guide the whole research process. The people being interviewed, and the nature of the research, will guide the nature of the interviewing process. For example, research with children may require the interview to be short and well structured and based somewhere the child feels comfortable (e.g. school or home). When interviewing adults, the process might benefit from allowing more time and being less structured in its approach to allow the interviewees' ideas and thoughts to be fully expressed and explored; although again, and depending on the nature of the research and the participants, the choice of venue for the research is important.

The philosophical basis of the study and the nature of the question to be asked will have the greatest bearing on the choice of interview type. Interviews may vary from short, structured surveys with precise, often **closed questions** (as you might find in a survey) through to unstructured and open questions that are primarily exploratory (as in phenomenology or grounded theory).

Concept summary: open and closed questions

Open questions are questions that do not suggest any sort of answer. They are a good way of starting a long and involved conversation. Open questions may start with phrases such as 'Tell me about …' or 'Describe to me …'. They focus on the what, why and how of human experience and understanding. They allow the respondent to take the lead in setting the direction in which the interview will go.

Closed questions are questions that suggest an answer or answers and invite only a limited range of responses. These may be 'yes', 'no' or factual answers such as one's age or town of residence. Closed questions may feature in later stages of a piece of research, and be used as a way of exploring the amount of agreement with an idea or theory a researcher has formed from earlier open questioning.

Activity 3.2   Research and finding out

Next time you are with a group of colleagues try asking different people one of the two following questions: 'How are you today?' or 'Are you alright?' Take note of the ways in which people respond to the two questions in terms of the fullness of their answers.

There are some possible answers at the end of the chapter.

Interviews usually take place in a private setting. The exact location depends on the nature of the interviews, the people being interviewed and other practical considerations. Often the interviews will take place in a room at a university or hospital, although for some purposes the home of the interviewee may be more appropriate. The COVID-19 pandemic has made the use of video calling more commonplace not only for personal chats, but for clinical interactions. Some researchers have started to use digital communication platforms for collecting data and go as far as to claim for some sensitive topics it may even be preferable (Howlett, 2021). This opens up a whole new world of possibilities within qualitative research which will need exploring over the coming years.

Qualitative interviews can last anything from half an hour up to about an hour and a half, although some may take much longer. If an interview is any shorter than this, it will fail to achieve satisfactory depth as there will not be enough time to probe. Longer interviews risk tiring both the interviewer and the interviewee, making them more likely to wander from the point. Again, the nature of the research, the interviewees and the questions that are being answered by the research determine the length of the interview, as will issues such as the availability of the researcher and the interviewee. Some methodologies, such as ethnography and bibliographic research, may require multiple interviews, the nature of which may be determined by the data collected in previous interviews; interviews are not always used as a one-off tool.

In qualitative research, interviews usually require the interviewer to go along with interviewees and to engage with what they are saying, rather than trying to control the interview (Sarantakos, 2012). Getting close to interviewees, probing and trying to gain a better understanding of what they are saying and the meaning they ascribe to a phenomenon gives qualitative interviewing the depth and richness we described earlier. This is in direct contrast to data collection methods used in quantitative research, where researchers must keep themselves as distant as possible from the research subjects while maintaining control over all aspects of the research process in the hope of avoiding the introduction of bias.

That said, while the interview needs to be 'open', it will require some direction so that the time the interviewer has with the interviewee is used to its maximum potential. Parahoo (2014) points out that in reality no interview can be entirely unstructured. This is logical since the interview has a purpose that will in some way guide the conversation to be about the issue being explored. This is somewhat like completing the paperwork when admitting someone to hospital; while you need to be able to explore the reasons they are there and their experience of symptoms of disease, you also need to complete the demographic details required.

All interviews should be recorded wherever possible, although a casual conversation in ethnography, for example, may not lend itself to this. The recording of the interview is generally important as it allows the researcher to capture word for word – **verbatim** – what the interviewee is saying. This means that there is no chance of the researcher forgetting something that has been said. Recording the interview also frees the researcher from having to take copious notes during the process, allowing them to concentrate on the content of the interview itself (Brinkmann and Kvale, 2014). The recording is then transcribed (that is, typed up) – again verbatim – to allow the researcher to read through the resulting transcript many times in order to identify the important issues raised.

It is crucial to establish the ground rules associated with an interview. These rules will cover anonymity and confidentiality. It is important to establish that the anonymity of the interviewee will be preserved throughout the research process, subject to the disclosures being legal and depending on local data protection rules. This will usually mean that the transcripts of the interview are given a code to identify the interviewee rather than being labelled with that person's name.

In health and social care, where issues of harm, potential harm or illegal behaviour are identified in an interview, it may be necessary to disclose these to someone in authority. The interviewee should understand this before the interview takes place, which can prove especially difficult where the researcher is engaged in ethnographical research (Delamont and Atkinson, 2018). It is never acceptable for nurse researchers to ignore legal or ethical issues that would cause concern in their day-to-day nursing practice just because they are engaged in research. For example, the disclosure of the abuse of a child or vulnerable adult or the threat of violence towards another person requires the researcher to bring the issue to the attention of the relevant authorities.

As well as recording the interview, it is important to write notes about the setting of the interview, the interviewee's body language and other non-verbal communications. Since the majority of human communication is non-verbal (Burgoon et al., 2016), these notes are an important tool in capturing the true meaning of the interview, and they provide context for the later analysis.

Activity 3.3   Research and finding out

Whenever you are next in a public place, take the time to look at the people around you and how they are interacting. Don't listen in to what people are saying; look at what they are

(Continued)

(Continued)

doing and pay special attention to their body language. Do you think they are happy, sad, bored, engrossed in what they are doing? What is it exactly about how they look which leads you to this conclusion? What does this tell you about the nature of human communication?

There are some possible answers at the end of the chapter.

Increasingly, researchers are using video recording to capture interviews. These offer the benefit not only of capturing verbal interaction but also the non-verbal aspects of an interaction. Pope and Mays (2020) identify video recording as acceptable to many research subjects, even when delicate issues are being discussed.

Ethical and practical issues associated with video recording must be taken into account. For example, it is difficult to exclude other people from a video if it is made in a public place, and some people will feel more vulnerable when filmed than when voice recorded, even if the filming is done in private. Again, the nature of the research question, the people being interviewed and practical considerations have to drive the decision about how any interview will be recorded.

Advantages

The key advantage of interviews is that they allow the exploration of a topic in more depth and have the potential to create *deep, rich* data. This is certainly true when they are compared to surveys and questionnaires, for example. Interviews allow interviewers to respond to and probe the responses that a participant has given and also to tailor the interview to what they hear (Sarantakos, 2012). In some instances, giving the participants sight of at least some of the questions prior to the interview will allow them to be better prepared and can help the process significantly.

As interviews are usually face to face, they allow the interviewer both to respond to and collect data, using field notes, about participants' body language during the questioning process. These data are helpful in establishing whether the interview subjects are happy to talk about the subject under investigation, and whether they appear to be answering in a truthful way, seem to be hiding something or are answering in a manner that they think the interviewer wants to hear (Tod, 2015). Having repeated access to visual cues is also one of the key advantages of video recording an interview and may contribute to their increase in popularity.

Interviews allow the interviewer to explain the meaning of a question or to rephrase it in a way that the interviewee understands if this is needed. This is a real strength over a self-completion questionnaire where respondents may either not understand a question or feel that the options available for answering do not represent their feelings or thoughts. Being able to explain a question also means that interviews can be used as a means of data collection where the interviewees have limited literacy skills (Tod, 2015).

Interviews are a very human process; they mimic day-to-day conversation, and in doing so can be made to feel comfortable for the interviewee, making them more likely to answer the questions they are asked. A skilled interviewer uses all the talents of a practised nurse in communicating with the interviewee, establishing a rapport and putting the interviewee at ease (something it is hard to do when not face to face).

Disadvantages

All of the disadvantages of interviews can be avoided by careful preparation and management of the process. The lack of prior experience of interviewing can be a major drawback: simple issues such as the phrasing of questions or tone of voice can have an enormous impact on how a research participant responds to a question. Although it is hard to get real-life experience of observing an interview, the novice researcher can read and listen to examples of interviews and learn some of the strategies in this way. The use of a **topic guide** or list of questions to be covered in the interview can help novice interviewers to achieve what they need from the interview process.

Interviews can be prone to a form of bias, where the person being interviewed answers questions in a way in which they think the questioner wants them answered (sometimes called the **Hawthorne effect**). This sort of problem is common in evaluation surveys (such as **rapid reviews** – discussed in Chapter 6) undertaken by researchers who are also part of the team that deliver the service being evaluated. An example of this may be the evaluation of a programme of study being carried out by the lecturers who deliver the programme or an evaluation of the benefits of a nurse-led clinic by the nurses who run it!

Interviews are often felt by novice researchers to be a quick and easy way of collecting data, but in fact they are very labour-intensive and require thought and preparation. Interviews also generally have to be typed up prior to analysis, adding further time to the process.

When using interviews as a data collection method, the process of knowing when enough data has been collected requires researchers to be aware of the point at which new data cease to emerge from interviews with new participants. This awareness can only come from being familiar with the content of all of the interviews as the data collection progresses. So the researcher now needs not only to conduct the interviews but also to transcribe them, or have them transcribed, and to keep their content fresh in his or her mind at all stages of the data collection process. Roulstin (2014, p306) states that, as a one-hour interview *may generate a 20-page transcript, interview projects may generate hundreds of pages of data.* This adds to the burden not only of producing the transcripts (which can be done by a professional transcriber) but in generating a lot of data for analysis. There is then the complication of adding in notes regarding body language at the appropriate part of the transcript, which again takes time and requires accuracy.

A further disadvantage of the interview process is that it is easy to deviate from the role of interviewer and to become the giver of information, present your own ideas and thoughts or engage in counselling activities. This is a common pitfall for many novice nurse researchers as they struggle to move from their clinical nursing role to that of a non-clinical researcher (Tod, 2015).

Powney and Watts (1987) make the ultimate observation about the disadvantages of interviews. They note that, as interviews are a way of collecting talk, and because talking is a dynamic interaction, this dynamic quality is lost when attempts are made to capture the talk – as in an interview. This gets to the nub of the problem with interview data: it is very much bound up with, and to, the time in which it was recorded. There is no doubt that the same question when asked in a different way (see Activity 3.2), on a different day or by a different person will elicit a different response. Talk, which is what interviews essentially are, belongs to the people involved, and it is hard to translate understanding and feeling from that moment into something that other people can fully understand.

Types of interviews

We have identified some of the major features all interviews share and looked at some of the strategies employed in interviewing. It is worth taking time now to look at some of the major groups of interview method that are used. This will help you gain insight into how they are undertaken. Although interviews are presented in the following sections as falling into one of two main types, in fact the degree of structure within the interview process is not that easily delineated. The degree of structure within any given study will lie somewhere on a continuum from completely structured to totally unstructured (Tod, 2015). Fully structured interviews which don't allow for the researcher to probe responses and therefore do not support the gathering of rich and deep data are better employed in quantitative data collection, which is discussed in Chapter 5.

Semi-structured interviews

Semi-structured interviews are interviews in which the key questions have been decided before the interview commences. In most cases the same questions are asked, but there is freedom within the interview protocol for the researcher to explore some of the answers given. The sequence of delivery of the questions varies from interviewee to interviewee and is guided by the responses the interviewees give. Adams (2010) identifies how the researcher undertaking semi-structured interviews needs to be agile enough to adapt the interview guide as they progress through their research.

Semi-structured interviews are, perhaps, the mostly widely used interview method in nursing research of whatever methodology because they have the dual advantage of having some structure while allowing for more in-depth probing of the answers a respondent gives. Semi-structured interviewing also allows the novice researcher the luxury of having a number of questions written down when starting the interview, thus allaying fears that the person might 'dry up' during the process.

Semi-structured interviews can be used with any of the qualitative research methodologies identified in Chapter 2. Because of the degree of structure within the process of a semi-structured interview, they cannot be seen as being as exploratory as unstructured interviews, and this may limit the interpretation of the findings of research using this particular method.

Because they do not have the same degree of detailed composition as structured interviews, semi-structured interviews can present the novice researcher with a bit of a challenge. Interviewers conducting semi-structured interviews still need to cover the majority, if not all, of the questions in the protocol while also responding to some of the issues and ideas raised by the interviewee; this can make them unpredictable in both content and length.

Unstructured interviews

Unstructured interviews are perhaps the most difficult to conduct and require some experience on the part of the researcher. They are only unstructured in so far as they do not start with lists of questions to be asked. Unstructured interviews often use topic guides, rather than questions. Topic guides are designed to allow interviewees to discuss their thoughts, feelings and perceptions on a topic as they see it. Unstructured interviews are exploratory and allow the researcher to gain insight into a topic without having formed any prior conceptions, as is generally the case with more structured interviews.

Unstructured interviews set out to gain an in-depth view of a topic from the point of view of the interviewee (the emic view) and therefore use probing questioning. Polit and Beck (2020) identify how unstructured interviews often start with what they call 'grand tour' questions which are open enough to allow the interviewee to start their answer as they see fit. The response to the grand tour questions allows the researcher to then ask more probing questions which are based on the interviewee's answer.

A key technique used in probing is to mirror back what the individual has said in order to ensure that it has been fully understood. Commonly, the interviewer will ask the interviewee questions such as, 'What did you mean when you said X?' and 'How did that make you feel?' Such questions are designed to gain more in-depth, rich, responses from the interviewee without providing any clues or guidance about what, if anything, it is that the interviewer expects to hear (again, see Activity 3.2).

Unstructured interviews are often used in studies that seek to gain an insight into a subject about which little is known. The data they produce may then be used in the design of subsequent studies or more structured interviews on the same topic area. Because of their usefulness in studying issues, ideas and experiences about which little is known, unstructured interviews are often used in more exploratory research such as phenomenology and grounded theory.

Activity 3.4   Research and finding out

When you are next in the clinical setting, spend some time talking to a patient in depth about that person's condition. Listen to what the patient says and use some of the techniques described above, like mirroring and probing, to gain a deeper understanding of the person's condition as they see it. Note how the patient responds to open questions and allow them to take the lead in how the discussion develops. Be careful to ensure you do not get out of your depth; discuss your intentions with your mentor before talking to a patient to make sure you choose the right patient and that there is support in place for both the patient and yourself should the need arise.

Focus groups

Focus groups are widely used to identify consensus feelings about the provision of services and the quality of products in both the public and private sector. Focus groups are a powerful and fairly rapid way of gaining insight into the collective views of a group of people. The researcher can access the views of many individuals in one setting during what is essentially a mass interview.

A well-run focus group will gain access to the views of all of the participants and will not only uncover pre-existing ideas and feelings, but also collect data on how the group's discussion and interaction changed the thoughts of the group, and those of the individual members of the group, about the topic under discussion. In this way they differ from interviews, because being involved in a focus group discussion can lead to the individuals changing their views because of what other people are saying. This change in views is not seen in the one-to-one interview and is something the researcher needs to take into account when deciding to use the focus group method.

The internet provides opportunities for researchers to undertake focus groups in the virtual environment. There are two key approaches to focus group data collection online. The first uses a simultaneous online chatroom-like format that allows people to participate in real time, while the other is more of a discussion board format, sometimes called asynchronous focus groups, where participants can log in and comment at a time and in a place convenient to them over a set period of time (Rivaz et al., 2019). Both of these methodologies are used to some effect by researchers who use social media platforms such as Twitter. There are several advantages with the accessibility of these types of internet-based studies, not least of which is that they are cheap and can recruit a lot of people with limited effort. They are, however, hard to moderate, and if the subject matter is evocative, it is hard to lend support to participants in a meaningful way if they become upset. Some of the more ephemeral media such as Twitter also do not lend themselves to collecting data which are either rich or deep.

Key features

In health and social care research, face-to-face focus groups usually consist of 6–12 people. Six is considered to be the minimum number of participants to enable a significant discussion, while 12 is close to the maximum that will allow the whole group to participate meaningfully in the discussion. The group is brought together because they all share some characteristic or experience that means they can usefully discuss the issue in question.

Focus group discussions are a good way of getting rich data about the views and opinions of the individuals involved. These views and opinions may evolve and change through the course of the focus group, allowing the individuals to develop a more in-depth understanding or opinion of the topic of interest, adding to the richness of the data collected. The use of the *group interview* allows participants to moderate each other's opinions and ideas through discussion, and may lead some of the participants to a point where they have a better understanding and more informed opinion of a topic than they would have if they had been interviewed alone. In many cases the effects of the group interaction are as interesting as the results of the focus group itself.

It is usual within focus group interviews to have one moderator, or facilitator, and one co-facilitator (also called an observer). The role of the facilitator is not to lead the discussion. It is to keep the participants focused on the topic under discussion, ask the generally unstructured and open questions (Creswell and Creswell, 2018) and try to engage all of the participants in the discussion. The observer is there to collect other data by observing the body language of the participants and taking notes about any patterns of behaviour exhibited during the focus group session. Observers are often also responsible for the process of video or audio recording the focus group.

Advantages

Key among the advantages of the focus group is that it allows people to be collectively interviewed in one place and at one time. While this usually does not remove the need for further focus groups or interviews as part of a study, it does mean that there is a rapid collection of data into which the researcher can tap. This means that focus groups have the potential to be a relatively inexpensive means of data collection.

In common with interview methods, focus groups are useful for collecting data from people who have limited literacy skills. The other interesting component of the focus group session is that the moderator can use the group to check their understanding of what the group has said while the group is still together. This process is sometimes called **member checking** and is a quality assurance tool used in research to establish the trustworthiness (or validity in quantitative research) of the interpretation the researcher has applied to the data collected (Pope and Mays, 2020). This means the participants can be involved in the data analysis and establishing the credibility of the findings. This can happen at the end of the focus group when the moderator sums up the discussion, brings together the ideas and themes raised and asks the group to confirm that the understanding of what they have said is correct. Alternatively, the moderator can collect together the themes and ask the participants to rank them in order of importance while they are still together. This means that, as well as data collection, the focus group can be used to start the analysis of the study.

Disadvantages

Carey and Asbury (2016) identify a number of potential problems with focus group interviewing, not least among which is getting everyone in the group involved with the discussion. There are always individuals within the group who are more confident and perhaps have more to say than the rest of the group, and their opinions then tend to rise to the forefront of the discussion, drawing others into their way of thinking, what Carey and Asbury (2016) call the 'band wagon effect'. Peterson and Barron (2007) suggest using sticky notes to collect people's ideas, either collectively or individually, before the focus group, and then using these as a stimulus to further discussion.

Acquiescence, or passive agreement, with the main group consensus can also be a problem within a focus group. There are two problems with a submissive group that tends to agree with what is being said because it is easier to do so than to challenge an opinion that appears to be popular. The first is that the consensus view may in fact not be the consensus; it may represent the views of the most vocal or powerful people in the group. The second problem is that the researcher also wants to hear and understand minority views and opinions in order to gain a more complete insight into the topic being studied.

The issues of acquiescence and non-involvement can both be designed out by carefully selecting focus groups that consist of people with similar degrees of power – within an organisation, for instance. A good example of keeping the power of the groups even would be using separate staff and patient focus groups to investigate feelings about changes to service provision within a hospital department.

There are also problems associated with the technology needed to capture all of the data produced in the focus group setting. While in an interview it is easy to place a voice recorder between the interviewer and interviewee, in the focus group setting this is not so easy. The recording of a group conversation is not only technically difficult, it can be difficult to decipher what is being said if more than one person talks at once. It may also be hard to catch the quieter members of the group. Focus groups conducted online may overcome many of these difficulties, especially where a chat forum methodology is used. These may exclude less literate individuals, however.

Transcription has the potential to change the meaning of what is said in either the focus group or interview setting. Although the interviewer should be able to ascribe meaning to comments made in the one-to-one setting, this can be quite hard to do in the focus group as different words have different meanings depending on the context and intonation used at the time of speaking. Writing up the body language and capturing the gestures and eye contact within the group is an important role of the co-facilitator as this allows such notes to be transposed on to (added to) the typed transcript of the focus group.

Observation

Observation may seem to be an unusual way of collecting data for research. Observation is something we associate with our day-to-day lives and also with the surveillance of patients in the clinical setting. Observation is, however, a powerful data collection method, and the ways in which it is undertaken, the amount of time it is undertaken for and the location in which the observation takes place have a large impact on the outputs from the research process. If interview methods are used to collect data about what people think, feel and understand, then observational data collection methods are used to collect data on what people do. There is sometimes a world of difference between what people say they do and what they actually do, and so observation as a method is used to capture data about very different questions to those which are served by interview methods.

Activity 3.5   Research and finding out

When you are next in the clinical setting observe the handwashing practices of the staff you are working with. All nurses and doctors will claim to wash their hands after patient contact, but if you observe them, is this really the case?

The process of data collection using observation is not unique to qualitative research. Observation is used in quantitative research, but there it tends to be more structured than in the qualitative methodologies. The things to be observed and noted are decided before the observation begins. What counts as an event for the observation is predetermined, and the data collected during the observation are ready for analysis as soon as the predetermined period and number of observations are complete. In quantitative research, things might be measured, for example, the surface area of a pressure sore, while in qualitative research no attempt is made to measure anything.

There are a number of forms that observation can take when collecting qualitative data. The most usual form is that of participant observation, which occurs in a number of guises and is discussed in more detail below.

Participant observation

Key features

Participant observation was introduced in Chapter 2 as a method associated primarily with ethnographic research. Participant observation is exactly what it says it is – the observations a researcher makes while participating in the life of a group. The first step in the participant observation process is the identification of the question or issue to be investigated, together with some thought about how the issues to be investigated might be observed. For example, if a researcher wants to understand what influences the activities of a group of nurses working in a given setting, the observer must first have some idea of what the activities they undertake are, and how often they undertake them, where and when. If the researcher were to ask the nurses what the influences were, the answer would be given to the question, 'What do nurses think the influences on their practice are?' If the researcher is engaged in participant observation, however, they can gain insights into 'the things which appear to influence nurses' practice'. These are very different starting points.

Concept summary: participant observation

Think about what you know about being a nurse. Consider the ideas and thoughts about what it is to be a nurse that you had before you started nursing as they were described to you by nurses you knew. Now compare these ideas to the reality of actually being a nurse, or student nurse. What you will notice is that your ideas of what it means to be a nurse have changed because of your experience and are somewhat different to the ideas you formed because of what people told you. They will have become more concrete and your understanding of the role of the nurse much firmer. This is similar to engaging in participant observation where participating in the life of a group increases understanding of not only what the group does but also the values and norms that the group has. In reality it probably differs greatly from what nurses told you about being a nurse before you joined the profession.

The next role for participant observers is to gain access to the area they want to observe. This is often via what are called gatekeepers – individuals who are part of the group the observer wants to study. Gatekeepers provide a means of accessing that group. In most cases in health and social care, this will mean being honest and open about what the research is about, although explaining the full extent of the purpose of the research may change behaviours within the group.

Once within the group, the observer must decide how to undertake the observations and record what they see and hear. This can include the use of tape recording, note taking or even video recording. You may think this sounds odd in relation to observation. In this context, however, observation means not only what the researcher sees, but also what they hear and what comes to the researcher during interviews with those being observed.

Some commentators suggest strategies and rules for participant observation that include: starting off passively; learning to fit into the group without actively seeking information; not getting too involved in what goes on; being careful to remain an observer rather than a participant; and avoiding being seen as an expert on any given topic.

Field notes from observations need to be written up as soon as possible after the event to ensure that the results of the observation are fresh in the mind of the observer. Stone Sunstein and Chiseri-Strater (2012) suggest that the following data are included in all field notes:

- date, time and place of observation;
- specific facts about what happens at the site of the observation;
- sensory impressions: sights, sounds, textures, smells, tastes;
- personal feelings about recording field notes;
- specific words, phrases, summaries of conversations and 'insider' language;
- questions about people, or behaviours, for future investigation;
- page numbers to keep the observations in order.

It is important to identify key informants, people who are willing to talk regularly and openly to the researcher about the topics under research. These key informants are useful sources of information, but they may have their own agendas and may not be representative of the group as a whole. Like gatekeepers, key informants may have their own agendas and power base within the group such that Coffey (2018) cautions that ethnographers should be cautious and treat their interactions with them sensitively and reflectively.

Statements and conversations that occur in a highly informal and voluntary manner may not be truly representative of what happens in the rest of the group or, indeed, when individuals are more aware that they are being observed or interviewed.

It is important for the observer to develop relationships with all the members of the group being observed. This may mean acting in ways similar to the group and adopting the language of the group. In many ways this is best achieved when the researcher/observer is also part of the group they are researching – for example, a nurse on the ward or in the clinic that is the subject of the research. Certainly, the behaviour of an individual one-to-one with the observer may vary widely from the individual's behaviour within the group. Differences in observed behaviours are worthy of note for the researcher and add to the context and interpretation of the observation. Table 3.1 sets out five dimensions of participant observation.

Role of observer	Portrayal of role to others	Portrayal of study purpose to others	Duration of research	Focus of observations
Full participant	Open	Open	Single	Narrow
Partial participant	Known to some	Partially disclosed	Several	Expanded
Onlooker	Hidden	Undisclosed/false explanation	Long-term	Very broad

Table 3.1 Five dimensions of participant observation

Source: adapted from Patton (1986).

Case study

In their ethnographic study of why registered nurses stay working, Ahlstedt et al. (2019) undertook four months of observations and 58 informal interviews including 10 registered nurses. They identified that nourishment, respect from colleagues, progress, positive work outcomes and increases in knowledge, and catalysts, times working alone and times working with others were key among the issues that made workplaces attractive to nurses.

As with much qualitative research, the analysis of the data collected is an ongoing process. The researcher notes the behaviours that occur and the circumstances under which they occur and creates preliminary ideas about what is being seen and why this occurs. These ideas will take into account the behaviours and activities seen and the context within which they occur. These explanations are then subject to review during subsequent observations and data collection such as interviews. These later observations may serve to support or challenge the ideas, or theories, initially generated.

Advantages

The main advantage of participant observation is that it accesses many forms of potential evidence. Unlike interviews and focus groups, which are restricted to what the people involved decide to tell the researcher, observations gather additional data about what researchers notice happening as well as what people tell them about their understanding of a phenomenon. Data from the observations have a richness and thickness that potentially surpass that of the interview because they have more context, making them more closely representative of what actually happens in a given situation.

Since observation, in the qualitative sense at least, is rarely a one-off event, the researcher has the opportunity not only to collect the initial data but also to verify whether these data are a true representation of what normally happens on subsequent occasions – this occurs as prolonged exposure to the researcher gives rise to familiarity and people revert to their usual patterns of behaviour (Coffey, 2018).

Participant observation, with its associated interviews and discussions, also has the capacity not only to record what people do but also to compare what they do to what they say they do. This duality of approach allows researchers to explore the interface between feelings, thought and reality in a way that may be meaningful to the study.

Disadvantages

The fact that one individual is ascribing meaning to events that they have witnessed means that the interpretation is open to subjectivity. There are masses of data – written, recorded and in other forms – to wade through. The analysis requires a large degree of selectivity on the part of the researcher, and it may not always be obvious which data to include and which not.

There are many ethical issues associated with data collection in participant observation, not least when the observations being undertaken are covert (hidden). This raises issues around consent and autonomy, especially in the clinical setting. Patients may come and go from the hospital ward, which may mean that they are not aware of, nor have consented to, being involved in data collection for a research project even if their role in the study is only passive.

Presenting and interpreting qualitative data

Readers of research cannot be present at all of the interviews, focus groups or observations, nor can they be expected to read through all of the data collected during the study. The closest they can get to understanding the meaning of the data collected is to read the data that the researcher has analysed, interpreted and presented. Not to present the data in this way would produce a massive amount of reading, which for the casual or, indeed, diligent reader will hold limited meaning anyway. This is because even reading the transcripts of an interview (which could be 20 pages long) does not provide an insight into the context of the conversation or of the body language that was being exhibited.

Because of the infeasibility of presenting all the rich and deep data collected within a study, certain processes and procedures need to be followed for collecting together all the data in a meaningful way for presentation to readers. This process involves identifying, whittling down and putting together the main points, observations or issues raised.

The argument was made earlier that this process is open to many problems, not least of which is sifting through the data collected. The large amounts of data and their subjective nature mean that a certain amount of trust has to be placed in the choices made by the researcher about which data to present and the final interpretations. Proficiency 1.8 of the Standards of Proficiency for Registered Nurses states that the registered nurse should 'demonstrate the knowledge, skills and ability to think critically when applying evidence and drawing on experience to make evidence informed decisions in all situations'. It is important, therefore, that readers of research understand some of the limitations of the research and analysis process and consider this when choosing when to 'apply relevant theory and research findings to their work'.

Key features

There are a number of different approaches to the analysis of qualitative data. It is beyond the scope of this text to explore these in detail (however, the further reading at the end of the chapter provides some sources which will enable you to do this); rather, it is important that the reader gains an insight into the overall strategies used and the reasons why they may be chosen.

As discussed in Chapter 1, the aim of qualitative research is to move from specific observations towards the generation of more general hypotheses. This process of theory generation usually occurs at the same time as the data are collected. This is quite unlike the process of data analysis that occurs in the quantitative methodologies, as we shall see in Chapter 5. Parahoo (2014) point out that analysis is a process that pervades the whole of the qualitative research process, both concurrently with data collection and following it.

The key data collected during qualitative research are the interview transcripts and the field notes, such as observations, made. The emphasis that is placed on every nuance of an interview, such as the silences, sighs and intonations, will vary according to the purpose of the research. For the most part, these relatively minor details are not an important part of data analysis. Rather, the researcher will seek to engage with the meaning of the words the interviewee says. For observations, again the exact nature of the research question will guide the data analysis process, with most qualitative researchers choosing not to narrow the focus of their research by applying a preconceived structure.

So we are left with a great deal of data in the form of words and observations that need to be narrowed down to a form that can be presented in a useful way. The key stage in this process of moving from broad observations to a general theory is to group similar data together in some meaningful way. This is more of a creative than a scientific process, and it requires a level of judgement on the part of the researcher.

According to O'Leary (2021), there are essentially six steps required to analyse qualitative data:

1. Identifying biases/noting overall impressions – if the researcher fails to do this, it is likely they will find whatever it is they want to find.
2. Reducing and coding into themes – requires the creation of categories and subcategories which may grow as the data are collected and analysed.

3. Searching for patterns and interconnections – themes will overlap and diverge, and it is important to identify these.

4. Mapping and building themes – using initial themes, continue building themes and sub themes and map any interconnections between these.

5. Building and verifying theories – this is the moment the data starts to make sense and the important ideas start to emerge after a lot of theme building and comparison work.

6. Drawing conclusions – this is about pulling the important threads from the data so it starts to make sense to other people reading it.

Reducing the raw data to something more manageable requires the reading and re-reading of the data. For interviews and focus groups this means reading the verbatim transcripts, and for observations this means reading both narrative and observation notes. Some programmes exist which can help researchers with the analysis of qualitative data. Such programmes, like NVivo, enable researchers to undertake content analysis of interviews and the like as the software searches for potential codes using key words and their synonyms.

During reading for manual data analysis, notes are made in the margins, identifying key issues, recurring words, their synonyms, and core ideas. In phenomenology these key issues are usually referred to as themes; in grounded theory they are codes; and in other qualitative research methods they come under various headings. Essentially, all qualitative analysis is about reading and identifying recurring ideas and notions from the participants.

The themes and codes identified in the first phase of the data analysis are then subjected to filtering down so that the important issues are identified and the less important removed. This filtration is not merely a matter of noting which issues occur most frequently within the various interviews, focus groups and observations, it is also a matter of noting those about which people feel most strongly. Other ideas may occur quite frequently but may not hold a lot of significance for the participants, which may be reflected in the emphasis the participants place upon them.

Identification of important themes is as much an art as a science, as was suggested earlier. The important themes within a qualitative enquiry will relate at least in part to the ideas contained within the initial question. There are a number of quality management strategies that can be used within qualitative research to ensure that this process is undertaken with a degree of certainty and credibility.

- Check with the focus group/interviewees that the issues they are trying to get across have been understood by reflecting them back to them at the time of the interview (a form of member checking).
- Send the identified themes/codes to the participants during the analysis to check if the key issues as they see them have been identified (a form of member checking).

- Use more than one person to analyse the data independently and compare notes later.
- Be reflexive throughout the process and be truthful about the influences and biases of the researchers and data analysts.
- Use direct quotes and/or observations to support the themes/codes identified, so readers can check the interpretations for themselves.
- Use qualitative data analysis software to analyse the data.

Depending on the methodology, once the themes and codes have been identified and whittled down to those that are the most important, it is time for the analyst to construct a theory or narrative account of the findings of the study, which lays bare the researcher's perception of what has been discovered. It is important that the research analysis goes beyond a mere description of the data collected, and that the analysis shows some relationship between the elements of the enquiry as identified during the study. As Doyle et al. (2020) point out, this process is as much about the ensuring the analysis reflects the aims of the study and the honest reflexivity of the researcher as it is about any the application of any consistent analytical method.

Going beyond a mere description requires that the analysis and presentation of the data manage to strike a balance between deliberate exploration of the data and open-mindedness (allowing the inductive process to lead where it will). In grounded theory this will lead the researcher to construct a theory about the issue under enquiry; in phenomenology this will result in the laying out of the key elements of the topic of interest (the essence of the phenomenon); in ethnography this will lead to an explanation of the group and how it works; and in a case study or generic qualitative research this is most likely to be a general discussion of what was found.

Once the data have been analysed, they need to be presented to readers in a manner that allows them not only to see what the analyst has seen, but also to believe it. The presentation should strike a balance between being descriptive and interpretative. There should be enough detail within the presentation to provide a deep insight into the key issues identified in the analysis. However, this needs to be tempered with enough focus, and the use of verbatim quotes, to present an argument or new theory that is believable.

The difficulty with relaying the findings of qualitative research is akin to the difficulty of trying to tell someone about an in-depth conversation you have had with someone else. The problems common to relaying the details of the conversation are about understanding what the other person has said, understanding what the individual did not say, looking for meaning and trying to express all of this to someone else who was not there.

Trustworthiness in qualitative research

The amount of trust that can be placed in a piece of qualitative research will depend to a great extent upon the quality of the processes that go into the data collection and the analysis (such as recording interviews and taking additional notes during a focus group). To a large degree, these rely on the description of both the data collection processes and analysis provided by the researcher that may then be judged by the reader. The idea of trustworthiness in qualitative research refers to a great extent to its ability to demonstrate both rigour (in the process of data collection; see above) and the relevance of the outcomes of the study (the quality of the product).

Henwood and Pidgeon (1992) suggest seven classic criteria for measuring good qualitative research. These criteria are associated with means of achieving sound research and as such provide a useful insight into how we might measure qualitative research quality.

Concept summary: qualitative research quality

1. *The importance of fit* – The themes from the analysis should fit the data: demonstrated by writing explicit accounts of how themes were derived.
2. *Integration of theory* – The relationship between the themes from the analysis and how they might be integrated (e.g. combined to generate a theory).
3. *Reflexivity* – The role of the researcher in the process is accounted for in the paper.
4. *Documentation* – An audit trail exists: the paper contains a comprehensive account of what was done and why decisions were made.
5. *Theoretical sampling and negative case analysis* – The researcher should continuously modify any emerging theory to include cases who do not fit the norm.
6. *Sensitivity to negotiated realities* – The researcher shows awareness of context, power and participant reactions within the process; especially true where there is a difference in interpretation between the research and the participants.
7. *Transferability* – Realistic suggestions about how the research findings might be usefully applied to help question and inform other related contexts of human experience.

(Adapted from Henwood and Pidgeon, 1992)

While many of these are a matter of judgement and personal interpretation, the fact that a researcher has taken the time to address elements of quality is a positive indication of intent. For novice readers, or doers, of qualitative research the key indicators of quality might well be considered to be the clarity with which the processes are explained and the degree to which the suggested findings are seen to fit (or perhaps coherently challenge) their pre-existing view of reality.

Chapter summary

This chapter has presented some of the methods used in the collection of data in qualitative research. We have seen that the collection of verbal data for qualitative research has

(Continued)

(Continued)

both great advantages and disadvantages, and that whether data are collected via interview or focus group, the process needs to be carefully managed. We have also noted that observation is an important tool of data collection in qualitative research, which involves the researchers themselves being tools of data collection. We have found, perhaps due to the in-depth and intrusive nature of the data collections, that qualitative research throws up myriad ethical and moral issues for the researcher which need addressing throughout the life of the study.

We have seen that qualitative research methods produce data that are very subjective in nature and that require the adoption of careful processes in order to add credibility and rigour to the qualitative research process. Key to the selection and execution of the data collection method within a qualitative enquiry is to understand the nature of the question that the research has set out to answer and what might be the best way of accessing that information.

We have seen that the nature of qualitative data collection is such that it is produced in large quantities that require careful collation and management. We have also seen that the process of data analysis in qualitative research involves extracting meaningful insights that contribute to the development of new understanding. This means that qualitative researchers have to make a number of decisions about how they will analyse and present the data they have collected, and be able to justify these decisions.

Activities: brief outline answers

Activity 3.1   Reflection (page 58)

Barriers that exist to good communication in the busy ward setting include the presence of other people and the inability of most ward areas to be able to provide privacy for such conversations to take place. Within the care setting, issues of time, the use of professional language and power relationships can also be barriers to good communication. The same issues exist in the research relationship.

Activity 3.2   Research and finding out (page 59)

When asking 'How are you?' you are asking an open question which invites people to be open and make a long response in which the person asked the question is given free rein to answer as fully as wished. The question 'Are you alright?' tends to suggest you want to hear a yes or no answer and so closes down the conversation, especially since most people see this as a cue to say 'yes'.

Activity 3.3   Research and finding out (page 61)

A great deal of human communication is non-verbal. That is, much communication is expressed in body language – for example, the way people hold their bodies, eye contact, smiling. In the case of verbally recorded interviews, it is not possible to capture this non-verbal communication unless the interviewer writes timed notes about posture and facial expressions at different points in the interview process.

Further reading

Brinkmann, S and Kvale, S (2014) *InterViews: Learning the Craft of Qualitative Research Interviewing* (3rd edn). London: Sage.

A comprehensive guide to interviews.

Carey, MA and Asbury J-O (2016) *Focus Group Research*. London: Routledge.

A comprehensive overview of this methodology.

Flick, U (2014) *The Sage Handbook of Qualitative Data Analysis*. London: Sage.

A comprehensive guide to qualitative data analysis.

Polit, DF and Beck, CT (2020) *Nursing Research: Generating and Assessing Evidence for Nursing Practice* (11th edn). London: Wolters Kluwer/Lippincott Williams & Wilkins.

Part 4 (especially 'Qualitative data analysis' and 'Trustworthiness and integrity in qualitative research') provides a quality discussion of data analysis and managing quality in qualitative research.

Useful websites

http://onlineqda.hud.ac.uk/ A useful introduction to qualitative data analysis.

www.ncrm.ac.uk/ It is worth looking at the resources page here at the National Centre for Research Methods.

http://sru.soc.surrey.ac.uk/SRU19.html An overview of focus group research.

www.socialresearchmethods.net/kb/index.php A comprehensive research textbook online.

Chapter 4
Overview of quantitative methodologies

Chapter aims

After reading this chapter, you will be able to:

- identify the main quantitative research methodologies used in health and social care;
- describe the type of research questions the different research methodologies can be used to answer;
- demonstrate awareness of how samples are chosen for quantitative studies;
- briefly describe the key methods of data collection used in each methodology.

Introduction

Epidemiology is the study of causes and consequences of disease in populations and is widely regarded as the major scientific discipline underpinning the practice of evidence-based medicine. For the most part, epidemiological studies are quantitative and employ fairly rigid and well-defined rules to ensure the accuracy of their findings. This chapter introduces you to the major quantitative methodologies (which are often termed epidemiological methodologies) and explains the theoretical and practical differences between them. It identifies the sorts of questions quantitative methodologies can be used to explore and the key characteristics of quantitative research. It then examines some of the main methodologies you will encounter in your nursing education and beyond. These are: quasi-experimental and experimental studies; randomised controlled trials (RCTs); cohort studies; case-control studies; and cross-sectional studies.

The chapter explores the strengths and weaknesses of each of these methodologies and considers which methodologies would be most suitable for different research questions. For example, when the research is seeking to prove **causality** (i.e. demonstrating cause and effect, as in exposure to asbestos causing mesothelioma or vaccination against the COVID-19 reducing the risk of disease), then only methodologies accepted to prove cause and effect (i.e. experimental and cohort studies) can be used. Other methodologies (case-control and cross-sectional) can be used to explore potential associations between a cause and effect (e.g. to explore a potential, but unproven, link between mobile phone use and brain tumours) or to measure the **prevalence** of an exposure or a disease (e.g. how many people with diabetes also have hypertension) but are not regarded as being of the right design to prove causality. The chapter also looks at the sampling methods (i.e. the ways in which study subjects are chosen) that can be used for each of the research methodologies identified.

The knowledge you gain from this chapter will enable you to identify quantitative research when you come across it in your own reading, and to evaluate and understand the methodologies used. It will also enable you to start thinking about how you could use these research methodologies to improve your own practice, especially after registration, as highlighted in Outcome 1.7 of the NMC Standards of Proficiency identified at the start of the chapter.

Case study

Dr John Snow undertook the first major **epidemiological** study in 1854. An outbreak of cholera (an infectious diarrhoeal illness) was killing a large number of people living in the Soho area of London, England. At that time, it was widely believed that miasmas (invisible and infected vapours carried on the wind) were the cause of ill health and disease; bacteria and viruses had not yet been discovered. Snow mapped the homes of the people affected by the disease and was drawn to believe (although, other than his own extensive observations, he had no scientific reason for believing this) that a water pump on Broad Street was the source of the outbreak. Snow persuaded the city authorities to remove the handle from the pump so no water could be drawn from it and the number of infections and deaths fell away rapidly.

Key characteristics of quantitative research

Quantitative research methodologies are used to answer questions that have a numerical element to them, or that set out to prove an association between two variables (cause and effect). Essentially, quantitative methodologies fall into one of two broad classifications: those that are **interventional** (or **experimental**) and those that are **observational** (**non-experimental**). Interventional studies seek to manipulate an **exposure** (the **independent variable**) in order to measure what effect it has on an outcome (the **dependent variable**) – for example, increasing education for people with diabetes (the independent variable or exposure) to improve their blood glucose levels (the dependent variable or **outcome**). Observational studies, on the other hand, seek to explore the associations between a naturally occurring independent variable (exposure) and a dependent variable (outcome) (Celentano and Szklo, 2019) or merely to quantify something in a population (e.g. how many student nurses smoke). This is because it is simply not always possible to be certain about what has caused something, often because there may be several potential causes contributing to an effect, some of which are known about and some of which are not, and it is necessary, therefore, to be more cautious about assigning a 'cause'. The terms

association and sometimes **correlation** (although this also has a strict research meaning, as you will see in the Glossary) are used instead. For example, there is an association between being obese and developing type 2 diabetes but the development of type 2 diabetes is also associated with a family history of the disease and other environmental and lifestyle factors.

Concept summary: cause and effect

A cause is simply something that has an effect. In quantitative research terminology it is common for a number of terms to be used for cause and effect, but essentially quantitative research is interested in causes (independent variables or exposures) and effects (dependent variables or outcomes). So we could describe the same event in one of three ways.

1.   A nosebleed (effect) may result from a punch to the nose (cause).
2.   A nosebleed (dependent variable) may result from a punch to the nose (independent variable).
3.   A nosebleed (outcome) may result from a punch to the nose (exposure).

The dependent variable is best thought of as occurring only if the independent variable has occurred. In this case the nosebleed is dependent on there having been a punch to the nose – if the punch had not been thrown, the nosebleed would not have happened. The independent variable is not affected by the dependent variable – obviously, a nosebleed will not cause a punch on the nose!

A small note of caution here: the dependent variable may sometimes arise as a result of the interplay of a number of independent variables, e.g. a genetic predisposition to having diabetes and being obese (independent variables) may sometimes need to be in play to give rise to a dependent variable, in this case developing diabetes. Similarly, while a particular independent variable may give rise, or contribute, to a dependent variable, effect, it may not be the only possible explanation. For example, some people develop diabetes in later life but are not obese or even overweight.

Understanding independent and dependent variables

This may all seem a bit complicated, but it is essentially just the terminology and rules that are applied to the study of cause and effect in healthcare. Understanding the nature and realities of cause and effect allows health professionals to intervene in a meaningful way in the lives of their patients. For example, having an understanding of the fact smoking is one of the causes of coronary heart disease, lung disease and cancer is useful for nurses who are seeking to engage in meaningful health promotion. Understanding that applying compression stockings after surgery reduces the occurrence of deep vein thromboses when compared to not using them equips nurses with information for practice that is worthwhile and potentially life-saving. Such evidence-based practice reflects a number of the NMC proficiencies.

The importance of quantitative research to nursing practice is clearly established, but the fact nurses undertake little in the way of quantitative research is of some concern. Establishing the benefits, or not, of some nursing practices would serve to advance nursing knowledge and practice and, more importantly, would be of great service to our patients. For example, using a randomised prospective study, Hoe and Nambiar (1985) famously demonstrated that the traditional nursing practice of shaving patients prior to surgery did not in fact reduce wound infection rates. Interestingly, a literature review by Bradshaw and Price (2007) demonstrated that the common practice of inserting rectal suppositories blunt end first – believed by many nurses to be evidence-based – relies on one questionnaire-based study published in *The Lancet* in 1991 that has not been subsequently verified! These examples identify the need for nurses both to understand the source of the ideas they read and to be able to critique the quality of the research which led to it before they use it to change their practice (more on this in Chapter 7).

There are a number of questions that quantitative research methods can be used to answer and, like qualitative methods, there are a number of issues the researcher has to take heed of before attempting to design a quantitative study. The key questions the methodologies explored in this chapter can answer are outlined in Table 4.1.

What is apparent from the table is that the sorts of questions quantitative methodologies can answer are highly interrelated. They tend towards asking questions about causes and effects and things that can be *measured* in one way or another, and they

Questions	Methodology
If *x* is done, what will happen? If *x* is done, how often will *y* happen?	Experiment/quasi-experiment/randomised controlled trial
If a person is exposed to *x*, will that person develop outcome (disease) *y*? Does exposure to *x* cause outcome *y*?	Cohort study
This individual has outcome *y*, what exposure *x* might have caused it?	Case-control study
In this group of people, how many have been exposed to *x* or have outcome *y*? What is the prevalence of *x* or *y* in this group?	Cross-sectional study
The data show that when *x* increases in the population so too does *y* – might they be associated?	Ecological study

Table 4.1   Questions that different quantitative methodologies can be used to answer

all have a *numerical* element to them. It is important to bear in mind, however, that if practice is to be established or changed on the basis of some quantitative research, it is imperative the correct methodology is chosen and properly applied. Table 4.1 gives an indication of the sorts of theoretical questions that can be answered using the different approaches. What follows will expand on these and give you a deeper insight into the questions and answers the different methodologies can be used to ask and answer, as well as the key features of these methodologies.

Activity 4.1   Reflection

Stop and think about the area that you are currently working in or your last placement. What type of nursing questions might quantitative research be used to answer about the sort of patient problems encountered or the care delivery undertaken there?

There are some possible answers at the end of the chapter.

Experimental and quasi-experimental research

Key features

The type of experiment described here does not relate to experiments that take place in the laboratory, but to ones that involve the researcher (or experimenter) examining the relationship between two variables – for example, does giving sucrose reduce the perception of pain in neonates? These experiments are carried out **prospectively** (that is, data are collected in real time and do not rely on memory or old notes) in an attempt to prove cause and effect. The reason any experiment is conducted is because there is genuine uncertainty about which treatment is best for the participants. This is called the *uncertainty principle* (described in Chapter 1), and 'best' in this context might be taken to mean cheapest, safest, most effective or easiest to use.

Observational studies (such as case-control and cross-sectional studies, which are studies that involve no intervention on the part of the researcher and are described later in this chapter) often lead to the generation of ideas for testing using experimental study designs. Sometimes it is hard to know which of two variables in an observational study caused the other to happen (if, indeed, they are at all related). A good example of this is the debate around the use of cold remedies. If patients take a cold remedy and get better within a few days, they may think that the remedy 'cured' their cold, even though it is likely they would have recovered equally well without taking the remedy. You might then ask the question, 'If the patient took the remedy and got better, does it matter whether the remedy worked or not?' This is a reasonable response, but what if the remedy were toxic, expensive or potentially dangerous? Many modern medicines and treatments are expensive and many have a host of side effects, and sometimes the medication or treatment has no real effect. The question therefore becomes, 'Why undertake treatments or give medications that are costly and have no benefits, or that are actually worse than doing nothing at all?'

The rise in antibiotic resistance is a consequence of the fact that antibiotics were, and often are, given to people unnecessarily. This demonstrates that there is a consequence to poor clinical practice that in turn is sometimes guided by poor research, poorly interpreted research or by ignoring the research.

Avoiding unnecessary expense and side effects provides one reason why it is important to undertake experimental studies into the usefulness of medications and other health-related interventions. Such questions require experimental approaches to answering them and demonstrate why these approaches are favoured in modern healthcare.

Case study

As an example of a clinical observation that was proven wrong by an RCT, the increased risk of cardiovascular events (especially stroke) in post-menopausal women taking hormone replacement therapy (HRT) was identified only during an RCT (an important experimental method, explained below) of HRT against a **placebo** (Writing Group for the Women's Health Initiative Investigators, 2002). Prior to this RCT, it had been thought that HRT actually protected women against cardiovascular events.

So experiments and quasi-experiments are types of research that are done to test cause and effect. The cause (independent variable) is manipulated, or introduced, by the researcher under carefully controlled conditions, and the effect (dependent variable) is then measured. Experiments and quasi-experiments are widely used to test the usefulness of: educational programmes in increasing understanding; clinical interventions in improving clinical outcomes; medicines in improving the management of disease; screening to identify disease; and the changing of methods of care delivery to improve the patient experience and satisfaction.

Hypotheses

When conducting an experiment it is good practice to start with a hypothesis. A hypothesis is literally an idea that is less than or below (*hypo*) a proposition or idea (*thesis*). That is, it is an idea that has yet to be tested or proven using the scientific method. The 'Concept summary' box shows the important characteristics of a hypothesis.

Concept summary: a hypothesis

Critical features of a hypothesis:

- suggest the relationship between the variables;
- identify the nature of the relationship;
- point to the research design to be used;
- indicate the population to be studied.

Hypotheses are often arrived at as the result of experience, clinical observation or observational research. Hypotheses remain theoretical until proven otherwise and even once 'proven' they remain open to further study; that is, something is only proven according to the ability of science at a given point in time (see Chapter 1, 'Concept summary: empiricism').

We have seen that in an experimental study the researcher manipulates one or more independent variables to see what happens to the dependent variable. In their simplest form (Figure 4.1) this means manipulating one independent variable in one group of participants and measuring the change in a dependent variable (often called a pre–post-test or before-and-after study).

Figure 4.1 A simple experimental design

Weaknesses

There are a number of issues with this type of study, not least that there is nothing to compare the intervention to and the outcome (reduced muscle pain in the example in Figure 4.1) might have occurred anyway if the person had just been left alone. Or perhaps it was the attention being paid to the individual that reduced the pain, and not the massage itself. The first issue is an example of what is called a **temporal effect**. This means it is an effect that occurs over time. The second issue is an example of the **placebo effect** – a perceived or measurable improvement in a person's condition that is not due to any active intervention but is, rather, the result of what is probably a subconscious psychological response to having an intervention (Murray, 2021). It is worth noting here that the placebo effect is not a bad thing: some commentators regard the placebo effect which arises from positive interactions between clinicians and patients to be at the core of the healing relationship (Kaptchuk and Miller, 2015).

There are two other issues with this type of simple experimental design: first, **regression to the mean** and second, **testing effects**. Regression to the mean occurs when individuals who have a variable measured for a second time in the post-test tend towards measurements that are more average than they were on the first occasion (e.g. satisfaction scores increase in those with initially low scores and decrease a little in those with initially high scores). This may happen regardless of the effects of the intervention (Walters et al., 2021). The other problem that may occur in this type of experiment results from the effects of the testing itself. For example, people subjected to a test involving an educational intervention may go away from the pre-test and find out about gaps in their knowledge, so when they are retested after the educational intervention their scores will rise because of the combined effects of the education and their own research. One way to overcome this is to do the pre- and post-tests a long way apart; the other is to introduce a **control arm** to the experiment (see RCTs, pages 91–96).

Quasi-experiments

The term quasi-experiment can be applied to the observation and measurement of changes that occur naturally (sometimes called natural experiments). In their natural experimental study of the impact of having a friend who was a teenage mother, Yakusheva and Fletcher (2015) demonstrated that the likelihood of teenage pregnancy diminished by 6 per cent in those teenagers who had a friend who had been pregnant and given birth. It may seem odd to think of this as an example of an experiment, because there is no manipulation of any variable by the researcher. However, when you consider that it might be impossible, or unethical, to undertake experiments on many subjects/issues, observing naturally occurring events provides a good window on the world of events which might otherwise be unethical to study.

Figure 4.2 represents a quasi-experimental design diagrammatically.

Surgery involved in screening   Surgery not involved in screening

Compare number of
diagnoses of diabetes

Figure 4.2 A quasi-experimental (natural experiment) design

A second form of quasi-experiment takes the methodology a little further. It examines two unrelated groups of people between which there is some difference in an independent variable. Measures are then taken of a suspected dependent variable, and the dependent variable for the two groups or **fixed cohorts** is compared. For example, in their quasi-experimental study of how likely a patient is to get a diagnosis of type 2 diabetes according to the level of participation of the GP practice in national screening initiatives, Palladino et al. (2017) demonstrated that patients in practices which actively engaged with national screening programmes were more likely to gain a diagnosis of type 2 diabetes than patients in those practices which were less engaged. This study is an example of a natural experiment comparing fixed cohorts – those practices whose engagement with national screening programmes was high, medium or low. The independent variable here is the level of engagement with the programme. Again, clearly this study might be considered to be unethical if undertaken as a prospective experiment, whereas, as is the case here, collecting data without changing existing practice is an acceptable means of assessing the impact on diagnosis of incident type 2 diabetes according to the level of practice engagement.

The third variation of the quasi-experiment is the pre–post-test study. In their natural experimental study of the impact of a community empowerment and health provider capacity building intervention on the uptake of antenatal, delivery and post-natal care and care practices of the newborn baby, Ekirapa-Kiracho et al. (2017) demonstrated improvements in all domains in the areas of Uganda where the intervention had been applied. In this form of quasi-experiment the subjects (or in this case, health districts) effectively become their own **control**. This design of a quasi-experiment is very useful in health policy research as it allows researchers to gauge the effectiveness of new healthcare policies on whole populations without disadvantaging any groups.

Quasi-experiments rely, therefore, on the measurement of unmanipulated independent and dependent variables. Because of this, and because there is no control over the environment in which the study takes place, there is a real danger that the outcomes of such experiments are affected by factors that are unknown to the researcher, and the results of such experiments therefore need to be treated with great caution. When working with such data, there is a real need to be certain that there is some plausibility to the associations being made – for example, health education changes health practices but increased availability of mobile phones does not!

Sampling in experimental and quasi-experimental research

The sample (that is, the individuals to be studied) chosen for an experimental study depends on the question posed in the hypothesis. Take the example of therapeutic massage and pain relief in Figure 4.1. First, it is important to define what constitutes pain and what part of the body is affected – let us say muscle pain in the thigh following sporting injury. There is a need to sample people from the population that exist with this condition, but there may well be a need to be more precise in defining the sample so that the effects of massage in a well-defined group are actually measured and described. The research sample may therefore consist of people experiencing a first soft-tissue injury of the leg with no broken bones. The outcome of the study would therefore apply only to people with the identified and described injury and not to other people experiencing a similar injury in their shoulder, say, or to people experiencing a second injury to the same thigh muscles or to those whose injury included a broken bone. Figure 4.3 gives a diagrammatic representation of sampling.

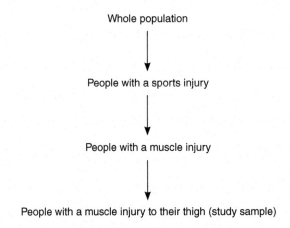

Figure 4.3 Sampling within an experimental study

Once these criteria are met and a large population (that is, people with the relevant injury) is identified, individuals for the study may then be chosen from that population – this is called the study sample. When the selection process gives everyone in the larger population the same chance of being in the study (so long as they meet the other criteria), this is called **probability sampling**, and when the sample size is big enough (often calculated using statistical formulae), a sample that is **representative** of the larger population has been produced.

Activity 4.2   Research and finding out

Look up and write down a definition of representativeness in research. Also look up the term generalisability and how this relates to representativeness. Thinking about what we have said about research influencing practice, why might generalisability be important?

There is a specimen answer given at the end of the chapter.

In a natural experiment, the sample for the study is the people who have experienced the phenomenon being researched. In the simple natural experiment they are the whole population affected by the change, while in the fixed cohorts design they are chosen because they come from one or other of the two groups under study. Studies which identify the impact on health at population level because of a health-modifying risk factor at that level – for example, the impact of deprivation on the risk of developing psychoses (Bhavsar et al., 2017) – are sometimes termed **ecological studies** as the risk of the outcome (psychoses) relates to the ecology (living conditions) of the people affected.

Methods used in data collection

Data collection in experimental and quasi-experimental studies depends on the exact question being investigated. The data collected can include: data about the independent variable, such as demographic data (e.g. age, gender and ethnicity), which may be collected from pre-existing sources such as databases or from individuals themselves, and data on a phenomenon (such as a sports injury or natural disaster), which may exist in patient notes, be collected from news sources or be collected especially for the study by interview or questionnaire (as with the data about the existence of post-natal depression by Palladino et al., 2017). Outcome (dependent variable) data may also be collected from existing records (as in the data used in the study by Bhavsar et al., 2017) or may be specially collected for the study using data collection methods such as interviews, questionnaires, physical examination or biological samples.

Randomised controlled trials
Key features

RCTs are widely considered to be the 'gold standard of proof' for a clinical intervention or the effectiveness of a medication. RCTs are conducted in a specific manner so that they are capable of answering a very specific question, or set of interrelated questions – for example: to determine the effects of vitamin D supplementation on the core symptoms of autism in children (Saad et al., 2018); to evaluate the impact on hemiplegic shoulder pain in people who have suffered a stroke of a modified wheelchair arm support (Pan et al., 2018); and the use of tranexamic acid in lower gastrointestinal haemorrhage (Smith et al., 2018). You may want to look up some of these in the library or online and explore how they have been undertaken.

RCTs are a very specific application of the experimental method identified above as they use techniques to explore the relationships between two (or often more) variables while maintaining direct control over other factors that may affect the **validity** and **reliability** of the findings.

Concept summary: validity and reliability

Validity refers to the ability of a methodology (or data collection technique) to measure what it is supposed to be measuring. For example, we know that a thermometer (if placed correctly for long enough) will measure temperature, but it is not easy to be certain that a questionnaire designed to measure quality of life does so, because it is not always easy to define what quality of life actually is.

Reliability refers to whether a method of data collection, or a measurement, will repeatedly give the same results if used by the same person more than once or by two or more people (so-called **inter-rater reliability**) when measuring the same phenomenon.

Because RCTs control many of the independent variables that a simple experiment does not, they have found favour as a source of evidence in medicine and, as the examples given above show, also in wider health and social care research. To understand why RCTs are so highly regarded it is worth paying attention to the key features of their design. The following discussion relates to the best possible design for an RCT: the 'gold standard'. However, it should be remembered that RCTs are very often conducted with human subjects, so there are good practical and ethical reasons why not all RCTs contain all of the features discussed below. An example of this is **equivalence studies**, where the current treatment for a condition is used instead of a placebo or **sham treatment** for comparison (see below). This is because it would be unethical not to treat people in the control arm when a treatment which is in general use already exists for the condition.

A control arm for a study provides the researchers with a group of individuals whose outcomes can be compared to the outcomes for the individuals in the study arm. People in the control arm of a study are treated in an identical manner to people in the study arm of the study minus the intervention or drug being tested. By doing this, the researcher can be sure that it is the intervention or the drug being researched that has caused the outcome of interest and not merely the fact that the individual has been involved in a research study, or indeed that behaviours have changed as a result of being in the study (see testing effects, earlier in the chapter).

Concept summary: control

The easiest way to understand why a control arm is important in a study is to consider what happens when a parent picks up a child who has fallen over and grazed her knee. The very act of picking up the child, saying 'there, there' and giving her a kiss is sufficient in most cases to make the child feel better. This is odd because no physical intervention has been

(Continued)

(Continued)

offered to make the pain go away; it is merely the attention which has the effect. Similarly, in a study of smoking cessation and the use of nicotine replacement therapy (NRT), failing to have a control group who see the nurse, get the advice but do not get the nicotine replacement patches or gum leaves us with a question at the end of the study: 'Is it the NRT which is having the impact, or the attention and information received while being part of the study?'

RCTs are always conducted in a prospective manner, which, as was discussed earlier in this chapter, means that data are collected in real time and do not rely on participant recall (which may lead to **recall bias**) or old notes or data. Prospective data collection also has the advantage of allowing researchers to collect the data they need rather than just that available to them after the event. This means both the type and quality of the data collected are better than that achieved using existing data sources (in most cases).

The study question is sometimes posed as a hypothesis, and sometimes as a **null hypothesis** (or the opposite of the outcome that the researchers expect to see and what the study sets out to disprove). The reasons for this relate to the statistics the study team will use and are not of great significance here. RCTs use one group on which a new intervention is tried and at least one other group on which the new intervention is not tried and with which the first group are compared. Both groups are treated in the same way, other than the intervention (the independent variable), so that the people conducting the RCT can demonstrate that the intervention, and nothing else, has caused the differences in outcomes (the dependent variable) between the groups. This is why they are an improvement on the simple experimental methodology described earlier. Figure 4.4 gives a diagrammatic representation of a simple RCT design.

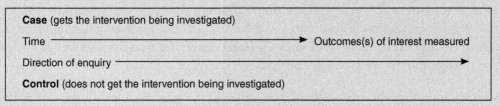

Figure 4.4 A simple randomised controlled trial design with one control group

Activity 4.3   Research and finding out

Consider the area in which you are working and some of the interventions you are involved with on a daily basis. Now consider what evidence might exist for these interventions and discuss these with your practice supervisor. Spend some time outside of work looking at whether you can find some evidence for the interventions. Do a search on a bibliographic database and/or look at the evidence contained in a NICE guideline and consider why much of this evidence is based on RCTS.

There are some possible answers at the end of the chapter.

Sampling in RCTs

The first problem with the above method, if we take it at face value, is to ensure the two groups (cases and controls) are alike at the start of the study. The simple solution to this issue might seem to be matching the two groups up for all the things that we can measure to make sure that this is the case. So, for example, if we wanted to test the usefulness of a new drug for lowering high blood cholesterol levels, we could get together a group of people who had high cholesterol and then split it into two groups. We could make sure that the two groups were evenly matched for age, gender, ethnicity, body mass index and whether they had high blood pressure or diabetes and claim that the two groups starting the study were identical. Indeed, if we accept that the issues identified are important in determining how people might respond to the drug this might seem reasonable. Some studies do closely match cases and controls for known variables, usually because there are few participants available for the research and sample sizes are small.

Matching cases and controls for all *known* variables is not always a good idea, since what this approach does not necessarily do is split the variables that we cannot see or measure – for instance, participant attitude and likely adherence to the trial regime, genetic make-up, social criteria and diet – evenly between the two groups. It is quite conceivable that these criteria are unevenly distributed among the participants and are affected by criteria we do not yet know about and lack the ability to measure. So the more usual way of dealing with the creation of the two groups is to allow them to be generated randomly, often by a computer or randomisation table.

The study starts with participants who all meet the inclusion criteria and are therefore similar in a number of ways. They are then randomly split into two groups so variables that can be seen and measured and variables that cannot be seen and measured are likely to be split evenly between the two groups (assuming that the number of participants included in the trial is large enough).

There is another reason why study staff do not split the participants into the two groups themselves: **selection bias**. Selection bias occurs when a researcher places a person in one arm of the study because they believe, perhaps subconsciously, that the person will benefit the most from the new intervention and/or that the individual is likely to show the new intervention in its best light.

Activity 4.4   Critical thinking

Imagine that you are involved in an RCT and are responsible for recruiting participants to the study and allocating them to be either cases or controls. Obviously you want the study to be a resounding success. What factors might affect the way in which you allocate people, assuming you have the choice about which arm of the study to put them into?

There are some possible answers at the end of the chapter.

The study is now at the point where the two groups have been determined and the new intervention is being applied in the case group and not in the control group. This gives rise to two new questions: 'Does it matter if participants can tell which group they are in?' and 'Does it matter if the researcher can tell which group each participant is in?'

Blinding in RCTs

The simple answer to these questions is that it is preferable that neither the participant nor the researcher can tell which group any individual participant is in. There are some good reasons for this. Participants are known to react differently if they know they are getting a new intervention. Returning to the cholesterol-lowering drug example, if the participants know they are on the cholesterol-lowering drug, they may choose to be less careful about their diet because, after all, they are getting the real thing; conversely, they may choose to increase their exercise and improve their diet because they want the study to work. Such **behavioural biases** (called the Hawthorne effect) will affect the confidence that can be placed in the study findings.

Activity 4.5   Reflection

Think back to your answers to Activity 3.2 in which you greeted some people by saying 'Are you alright?' and others by saying 'How are you today?' You will recall we observed that people will respond in the way they believe you want to hear. In what way might similar additional behavioural biases be introduced to an RCT if the researchers know what group the participants are allocated to?

There is an explanation of this activity at the end of the chapter.

If researchers know what arm of a study a participant is in, this too may change their behaviour, either consciously or subconsciously, again because they want to be part of something successful. This may mean that in a trial of a new wound dressing they report improved wound healing for a new dressing; or in the cholesterol-lowering example, they may give the intervention group more education about diet, exercise and smoking cessation than they give to the control group. It is also always possible that their interactions and questioning about symptoms will not be the same between groups.

To avoid behavioural biases, gold-standard RCTs blind both the participants and researchers to which arm of the study each participant is on. This **blinding** (now sometimes called **masking**) is usually achieved by the use of a placebo in a drug trial or a sham intervention in a trial of a treatment. A placebo is a drug that looks exactly like the drug being trialled, but that does not contain the active drug. Sham interventions are harder to provide – for instance, it is hard to pretend to give a therapeutic massage or to hide which wound dressing is being used. One way round this is for the person delivering the intervention and the person recording the effectiveness of the intervention to be different so that prior knowledge of what treatment a patient is receiving does not bias the measurements being taken.

Methods used for data collection

RCTs use a number of methods for collecting the study data. These methods include clinical and non-clinical measurements (e.g. blood cholesterol levels, wound-healing rates, participant satisfaction and quality-of-life data). The methods used for data collection are determined by the outcomes that the study is measuring. All methods of data collection need to measure the variables concerned both accurately and clearly (Parahoo, 2014). This means that when designing research it is important to define what is being measured as well as how it is being measured, by whom and when, and to ensure that all researchers involved in the study (which may be taking place across many different sites, for example) follow precisely the same protocol (thus increasing the inter-rater reliability of the study).

Many RCTs collect data on more than one outcome, so they may use clinical measures and questionnaires simultaneously to obtain data to answer the research question. In order to maintain blinding, the results of clinical tests such as cholesterol levels are not known to either the researcher or the participant but are surveyed by a monitoring team that also has responsibility for making sure that the participants in a study are kept safe and that it is stopped if there are any unforeseen adverse consequences. Monitors may also stop a study early if the proof required of it is derived early, so-called 'stopping early for benefit', although doing this does risk the study's findings remaining subject to question.

Many of the questionnaires used in RCTs and other forms of quantitative research have been previously validated, that is, they have been tested on many occasions in several groups of individuals to make sure that the questions they contain gain a true picture of what people actually think or feel about an issue. A common example of such a questionnaire is the Short Form 36 (SF36), which is used to measure an individual's health and well-being as that person sees it (**https://orthotoolkit.com/sf-36/**) and has been validated in different languages among people with different health conditions.

Activity 4.6   Research and finding out

Go online and identify some pre-validated questionnaires which might be used by researchers. Such questionnaires might ask questions about a person's general health, mental health, mobility, quality of life or social functioning. Read up about the questionnaires, how they were designed and validated and what they might be used for. Examples include: the Hospital Anxiety and Depressions Scale (HADS); the World Health Organization Quality of Life (WHOQOL); and the Social Functioning Questionnaire (SFQ).

Cohort studies

Key features

Cohort studies are usually prospective and follow a predetermined group of individuals through time and measure the **incidence** of predetermined outcomes. For example, cohort studies might be used to follow a group of workers in the asbestos industry for a period of years to determine the incidence of mesothelioma (a type of lung cancer associated with exposure to asbestos) in that group (Nicholson et al., 1982). The purpose of cohort studies is to link an exposure (independent variable or cause – in this case, asbestos) with an outcome (dependent variable or effect – in this case, mesothelioma). Cohort studies are said to be able to determine the causality of disease, that is, they are able to link exposure to a certain independent variable with a disease being researched.

Concept summary: cohorts

To understand the concept of cohorts, think about the people with whom you trained or are training. They are your training cohort. Because you are training in a caring profession, you will share some characteristics: you are all likely to like people, be caring and have broadly similar values. Because you are training or have trained together, you share similar skills because you have been exposed to similar classroom and clinical situations. As you are a cohort, it is likely therefore you will have some shared outcomes that result from your shared exposures.

Unlike the experimental study designs discussed earlier, cohort studies do not involve an intervention on the part of the researcher – they are purely observational. It is the fact these studies are undertaken prospectively and that they explain the biological reasons for the disease outcome that makes them able to determine the causality of disease. Figure 4.5 gives a diagrammatic representation of a simple cohort study.

Figure 4.5 A simple cohort study design with one control group

What you will notice from Figure 4.5 is that some people get the disease even though they were not thought to be exposed to a cause of the disease. There are two main reasons for this. First, disease may have more than one cause and so the cohort study provides insight into how much is actually caused by the exposure under investigation rather than other environmental or lifestyle exposures. Second, people are often exposed to things they do not know about – for example, they may be exposed to asbestos in an old house or place of work and, as is commonly recognised now, through handling and washing the overalls of a spouse who works directly with asbestos.

Some cohort studies are **retrospective** (that is, they look back in time) and try to collect data about an exposure (a potential cause of disease) and relate it to an outcome (often a disease). However, less faith is placed in the outcomes of these types of studies because they are not prospective and so rely on the recall of participants for things such as dietary or smoking history. This may cause recall bias, which leads to questions about whether the study does indeed demonstrate what it claims to demonstrate. Althubaiti (2016) gives the example of people having erroneous recollections in relation to their dietary intake when they have developed a diet related disease. Such recollections might cause the association between diet and ill health to be underestimated within the research.

As well as cohort studies that follow well-defined groups of people over a period of time to collect data on the incidence of a particular disease (as in the asbestos and mesothelioma example), there is another form of prospective cohort study design that follows people over a period of time and collects data about their lifestyle, blood pressure, diet and working lives (exposures or independent variables) as well as collecting data about the development of disease and ill health (outcomes or dependent variables) in the cohort. The data collected on exposure, and indeed non-exposure, are then compared to data on outcomes, or not, in the cohort. Inferences are then made about the causes of disease and ill health. The benefit of this form of cohort study is that it does not have to start with any preconceptions and is therefore useful in identifying causes of disease that had not previously been thought of.

A number of famous cohort studies have given useful insights into what lifestyle choices, jobs and medication regimes give rise to increased likelihood of disease. Perhaps the most interesting studies for nurses are the massive and very productive Nurses' Health Studies that are taking place in the USA (see case study).

Case study

The Nurses' Health Study cohort research project (NHS I) was started in 1976 and its scope and cohort size were further expanded in 1989. In 1976 the study enrolled married registered nurses aged 30–55 who lived in the 11 US states where the state nursing boards had agreed to supply the nurses' names and addresses. Of the 170,000 nurses initially approached,

(Continued)

(Continued)

approximately 122,000 nurses responded. Every two years since then, all members of the cohort have received a follow-up questionnaire regarding diseases and health-related topics, including smoking, hormone use and menopausal status. Every four years since 1980, the cohort have also received questions relating to their dietary habits, and since 1990 questions about quality of life have been added. Response rates to the questionnaires have been high, at about 90 per cent, throughout its life (**www.channing.harvard.edu/nhs**).

A second study (NHS II) was started in 1989 with younger participants – aged 25–42 – in order to study emerging areas of interest such as contraception use, diet and more lifestyle data. The cohort for this study is somewhat smaller, at around 117,000 participants.

NHS III is the newest study: it is web-based and started to roll out in 2008, again to a younger generation of nurses, for the first-time including men as well as Canadian nurses. NHS III is collecting broader data than I and II to include environmental as well as mental health issues.

What is interesting about these studies is that they have taken an informed set of professionals and collected data in real time over many years. If an individual nurse enrolled in 1976 and is still participating in the study – as many are – then, to date, there are over 40 years of data relating to the one individual. Given the size of the initial cohort, this means that NHS I has data relating to over 4.5 million years of nurses' lives, the things they are exposed to and the outcomes and diseases these might cause. To date, these studies have produced, and are still producing, many hundreds of research papers relating to disease risk factors for women. Some of the key findings from NHS I and NHS II are shown in Table 4.2. You may find that exploring the website for this study gives you some understanding of the nature of these types of study.

* Birth control pills do not increase non-smoking women's risk of heart disease
* Women who take oral contraceptives for more than five years have less than half the risk of ovarian cancer than women who have never used birth control pills
* Women who take oestrogen after menopause decrease their risk of heart disease, but raise their risk of developing breast cancer
* Increased dietary calcium intake among post-menopausal women is not protective against fractures of the hip and wrist, although a positive relationship has been observed between protein intake and risk of fractures
* A diet rich in red meat raises the risk of colon cancer
* Women who drink moderate amounts of alcohol (one to three drinks per week) cut their risk of heart attack in half, but increase their risk of breast cancer by one-third
* Limiting fat intake and eating more high-fibre foods does not reduce a woman's risk of breast cancer
* Women who have taken multi-vitamin supplements that contain folic acid have a 75 per cent reduced risk of colon cancer.

Table 4.2   Some of the major findings of the Nurses' Health Studies

Source: **www.channing.harvard.edu/nhs**

Activity 4.7   Research and finding out

Many good-quality cohort studies have contributed widely to our understanding of the causes of disease, whether those causes relate to lifestyle, diet, exercise, occupation or something else. Go online and find three or four other cohort studies and identify the key findings they have demonstrated which have contributed to our understanding of factors contributing to good health and disease. A couple of examples which are of most interest include: Whitehall I and II (ongoing) and the British Doctors Study (analysis of which is still ongoing).

Sampling in cohort studies

The sample selected for a cohort study is determined by the questions that the study sets out to answer. So if the study is interested in specific outcomes for a specific group (such as individuals who work with asbestos), then people who meet the criteria of interest constitute the study group or sample. If, however, the study is interested in determining several outcomes, especially where there is no suspicion of a particular disease in a group, then a more general group is chosen and followed up for a period of time, measuring a range of exposures and outcomes to see what arises (the Nurses' Health Studies would fall into this category).

As with RCTs, there remains the need for a comparison group so it is possible to compare exposure in one group to non-exposure in the other and thus determine the extent to which the outcome of interest is caused by the exposure (demonstrating causality).

There are many issues relating to how and who is selected to be in the comparison group, as there is a need to keep the two groups as alike as possible in order that the one thing that is different between the groups can be said to be the exposure that has caused the outcome. In studies such as the Nurses' Health Studies, this is achieved by studying a large homogeneous (largely similar) group of nurses of similar ages and, when an outcome of interest arises, comparing the data on exposures between those who have the outcome (or disease) of interest and those who do not.

In more specific cohort studies, such as the asbestos workers example, the comparison group would be drawn from people who are largely similar to the group being investigated except they are not exposed to the potential cause being investigated. So a comparison group for people who work with asbestos might include other workers in the same factory, or workers in similar jobs who live in the same community and have broadly similar lifestyles to the group under study.

Methods used for data collection

The most frequently used data collection method in cohort studies is self-completion questionnaires. The use of self-completion questionnaires is driven by the fact that these studies are so large and take place over such long periods of time that individual visits, or data collection by study staff, would be very expensive and time consuming. Some studies collect additional data from some participants for analysis of subgroups or because there is a suspicion the extra data will yield some useful results. For example, for various purposes the NHS I study has collected toenail clippings (to examine mineral content) as well as blood samples (usually more than one sample, and some years apart) from many thousands of participants.

As with the RCT, some of the questionnaires used are previously validated while other questions and questionnaires are designed specifically for the study.

Case-control studies
Key features

Case-control studies are cheap and easy to do when compared with other quantitative research methods (they are not related to, nor do they answer similar questions to, RCTs). Case-control studies are backward looking (retrospective). They study people with an outcome (or disease – the dependent variable) of interest and try to determine past exposures (the independent variable) to things that might have caused the disease (Celentano and Szklo, 2019), or might predict the occurrence of an outcome. For example, in their study of suicides among people with a diagnosis of psychiatric illness, Chen et al. (2018) identified that individuals who also had a disease of the pancreas were more likely to have taken their own lives than those who did not have pancreatic disease; Broberg et al. (2018) demonstrated in their case-control study that women who had less disposable income, with lower education attainment or who were not cohabiting, were less likely to take up cervical screening; and Abete et al. (2018) demonstrated a link between low physical activity, smoking, and taking a diet with a high inflammatory potential and an increased risk of stroke.

Case-control studies cannot be used to prove causality because they do not collect data in a prospective manner and so there are many issues relating to **confounding** and bias that may affect the quality of the data they produce. People with the disease in question may recall exposure to the causal agent better than people without the disease because they have thought about it. As explained earlier, this is called recall bias. A case-control study must have a hypothesis, or hypotheses, as this makes the design of the study easier and more understandable to people who might read it. Figure 4.6 gives a diagrammatic representation of a case-control study.

Figure 4.6   A case-control study

Concept summary: confounding

Confounding occurs when alternative explanations for an outcome in a study are not accounted for. Confounding variables are always independently associated with both the exposure and the outcome being measured. For example, an increased risk of coronary heart disease (the outcome) is attributable to both smoking (the exposure/independent variable being studied) and high alcohol consumption (an exposure/independent variable not being studied); however, smokers are known to drink more than non-smokers generally so smoking and drinking are independently associated both with each other and the outcome of interest, coronary heart disease.

In the mesothelioma cohort study, if the control group used was very different from the study group – for example, if it was composed of office workers who as such are less likely to smoke than manual workers who work with asbestos – then smoking might be responsible for making the manual workers more susceptible to mesothelioma. So the risk of getting mesothelioma from exposure to asbestos might be overestimated if the levels of smoking in the two groups were not accounted for.

Sampling in case-control studies

The sample for a case-control study is taken by selecting people who have an outcome of interest – in our examples, have taken their own lives, have not taken up cervical screening and have had a stroke – and matching them with appropriately matched individuals who do not have the outcome of interest. Cases need to be well defined. It is not enough, for instance, to define your sample as 'people with hypertension' (high blood pressure); it is better to state what is meant by high blood pressure (e.g. 'greater than 150/85 mmHg on three consecutive occasions'). It is also important to define where the cases are from (their source), because this provides information about how representative they are of all people with the outcome of interest. At its simplest, all cases of liver cancer in one hospital in the UK may not be representative of all cases of liver cancer, especially if the hospital is in an area of high unemployment or social deprivation, for example. When subjects are drawn from prevalent cases (rather than incident ones) they may be different from the whole population of people with the disease. This may be because prevalence of the disease relies on people surviving with it, whereas using incident cases does not.

Concept summary: prevalent cases

Prevalent cases are people with a disease (or other outcome of interest) at a given point in time. Incident cases are new cases of a disease (or other outcome of interest) occurring during the course of the research study. So prevalent cases are existing cases and incident cases are new cases. The important issue is survival: if a study uses prevalent cases, but the disease has a high early **mortality rate**, then prevalent cases may not represent the majority of people who get the disease because many of them will have died.

Disease duration also affects the choice of prevalent or incident cases. If one is studying an outbreak of food poisoning, then one would study incident cases as the illness is short-lived. But when researching chronic diseases (such as diabetes or chronic kidney disease), the choice of prevalent or incident cases is influenced more by the research question than the disease duration.

Choosing controls for case-control studies is as much a matter of judgement as it is of science. Controls need to be chosen with care. If the aim of the study is to compare like with like, then the controls need to be very similar – in all respects other than not having the disease – to the case population.

A good example that demonstrates the need for good judgement is the study of a disease that is related to alcohol. If the cases are all people who have been admitted to hospital with alcohol-related liver disease, it may seem sensible to compare them to other people in the hospital at the same time who are of the same gender and age. There is a problem with this, however, since people who have alcohol-related accidents or alcohol-related diseases are admitted to hospital more often than people in the population as a whole with the same gender and age. So a control group chosen like this would be less like the general population from which the cases are drawn than if it was drawn from the general population.

When next in practice, you may want to take note of the number of patients you see who smoke or have a history of excessive alcohol use. What you will note is that the percentage who smoke or who drink to excess is greater than the percentage of people in the general population who drink or smoke.

Methods used for data collection

Data collection for case-control studies is usually undertaken by studying medical, nursing and other documentary records, by interviewing (the cases and controls or their relatives) and by taking or using existing, biological samples. One of the major problems with case-control studies – and a good reason why they are generally used to generate hypotheses that are later tested in prospective studies – is that they often rely on participant recall (which is open to charges of recall bias). The other issue of note is that the use of retrospective data does not allow the researcher any control over what data are collected or quality. This means there can be issues with both validity and reliability.

Cross-sectional studies

Key features

Cross-sectional studies are used to research the prevalence of an outcome or exposure in a given group. They are very common in healthcare research and are quick, cheap and easy to conduct. Cross-sectional studies allow researchers to generate hypotheses that can be tested using other quantitative methods such as RCTs and cohort studies.

Cross-sectional studies often use survey methods to find out any number of things, including demographic data, the presence or absence of disease, people's opinions and the way in which people plan to vote. It is usual practice for universities to collect data on students' opinions of the modules they are studying; this is a simple cross-sectional study usually undertaken for quality monitoring (audit) purposes.

Since data on exposures and outcomes are collected simultaneously, cross-sectional studies are not good at showing the sequence of events (the **temporal sequence**). For example, a cross-sectional study of mental illness and unemployment would be hard to interpret since it is likely that mental illness is both a cause and effect of being unemployed. Because of this they are the weakest of the epidemiological study designs discussed in this chapter.

Cross-sectional studies usually measure one of two types of prevalence: **point prevalence** ('Do you have a headache at the moment?') and **period prevalence** ('Have you had a headache in the last week?'). For chronic diseases (diseases that last a long time, such as asthma or diabetes) there is little difference between the two measures of prevalence, while for short-lived diseases (such as a cold or a headache) the two may be vastly different.

A cross-sectional study is essentially a snapshot of a phenomenon at a point in time and cannot, therefore, be used to demonstrate the incidence of an exposure or an outcome, unlike the prospective methods discussed earlier. Unless they are focused on high-risk groups, cross-sectional studies are not very useful for studying rare diseases. Cross-sectional studies can be useful for planning the delivery of a service and for estimating future need.

Some cross-sectional studies collect data on two phenomena of interest and examine whether there is an association (or correlation) between the two, although, because cross-sectional studies are not, usually, longitudinal, they are not able to demonstrate true cause and effect. One such study by Saga et al. (2015) sought to examine the prevalence of urinary and faecal incontinence in nursing home residents and what characteristics might make residents more likely to suffer from these.

Sampling in cross-sectional studies

The sample for a cross-sectional study is usually drawn from a population in which the exposures or outcomes of interest are known to be fairly prevalent. For example, Ellis and Cairns (2001) studied the period prevalence of renal disease among older people with hypertension and/or diabetes in two GP practices. The purpose of this study was to ascertain the prevalence of early renal disease in order to inform the debate about whether screening for renal disease among this population was a worthwhile exercise.

Methods used for data collection

Data for cross-sectional studies are often drawn from pre-existing data, such as blood test results, data held on hospital or GP databases, or data held by local authorities. Such data may be supplemented during the course of a study by taking biological samples, by using questionnaires or by conducting structured interviews. Again, as much of this data is collected outside of the study protocol it is subject to quality issues like validity, reliability and bias.

Chapter summary

This chapter has described the main quantitative methodologies used in healthcare research. It has identified that the choice of study design is influenced by a number of issues that include the nature of the question being asked, whether the study is attempting to show cause and effect (experimental designs and cohort studies) or whether it is interested in looking for potential associations (case-control) or merely measuring the prevalence of a phenomenon (cross-sectional studies).

We have seen that the samples used in various studies have to be carefully chosen and described in order to maintain the validity of the study and that various data collection methods have to be used consistently (reliably) in order to generate the findings for a given research methodology.

The following chapter describes and explores in more detail the data collection methods used in quantitative research and when they might be used, as well as their strengths and weaknesses. It shows some of the methods used for describing the data found during a quantitative study and some of the statistical tests used to generate findings.

Activities: brief outline answers

Activity 4.1   Reflection (page 85)

Here are some types of questions that quantitative research might be used to answer.

- How can nurses effectively measure pain and the effects of analgesia?
- Is patient mortality linked to the nurse–patient ratio on the ward?
- Does using dressing a result in less wound infections for patients undergoing knee replacement?
- Does home birth result in fewer complication for the mother than hospital birth?

Activity 4.2   Research and finding out (page 90)

Representativeness is the extent to which the study sample is similar to the general population from which it is drawn for important variables (e.g. gender, age, ethnicity). The more representative a study sample, the more likely that the findings of the study hold true for the general population (generalisability). High levels of representativeness and generalisability mean a fair degree of faith can be placed in applying the findings of the study to the general population, that is, they make good evidence for informing practice.

Activity 4.3   Research and finding out (page 93)

RCTs are used to determine cause and effect and may be used to demonstrate the effectiveness of a drug or a therapeutic intervention. They are also used to compare new and old drugs or usual interventions. Example investigations might include the following.

- Does patient-controlled analgesia improve patient satisfaction with knee replacement surgery when compared to four-hourly injections?
- Do children admitted to the emergency department with an exacerbation of asthma respond as well to a reservoir spacing device as they do to a nebuliser?
- Do patients with arthritis report better mobility with the new drug x than they did with the old drug y?

Problems with undertaking RCTs in the practice setting include time, making sure everyone follows the trial protocol and procedures properly, and keeping accurate records of interventions. You may discover that the findings of the RCT you have located are embedded in practice; if they are not, discuss with your practice supervisor why this might not be the case – for example, it is too expensive, the RCT does not reflect the findings of other studies, NICE have adopted other protocols.

Activity 4.4   Critical thinking (page 94)

Any researcher might be tempted to put the sickest participants into the cases arm (group) as they might show the best response. It is also possible, depending on the study, that putting the least sick participants into the cases arm might achieve the best result. There might also be the temptation to put into the cases group the most articulate participants or those considered most likely to comply or try hardest to achieve the goals of the study. Such choices may be conscious decisions or made purely subconsciously. Either way, they mean that the study would not be comparing like with like.

Activity 4.5   Reflection (page 95)

Most people like to be liked; one way that people ensure that they are liked is to behave in a way that they think you want them to behave. When you say 'Are you alright?', what they are hearing is, 'I want you to say that you are alright', but when you say 'How are you today?' they hear an open question that has no suggested response, so they feel more able to respond by saying how they actually feel. This is similar to the Hawthorne effect in that people are responding to what they think you want to hear, rather than saying what they actually want to say. If researchers know what group a participant is allocated to in a study, this may lead to them treating people in the two arms differently and asking the same questions in different ways, or in a different tone, when interacting with participants in the different groups.

Further reading

Gerrish, K and Lathlean, J (eds) (2015) *The Research Process in Nursing* (7th edn). Oxford: Wiley-Blackwell.

See Chapter 17 on experimental research, Chapter 18 on survey methods and Chapter 30 on questionnaire design and use.

Celentano, M and Szklo, DD (2019) *Gordis Epidemiology*. Philadelphia: Elsevier.

A classic and very accessible guide to all epidemiology, especially the research designs.

Parahoo, K (2014) *Nursing Research: Principles, Process and Issues* (3rd edn). London: Palgrave Macmillan.

See Chapter 3 on quantitative designs, Chapter 11 on experimental design and Chapter 13 on questionnaires.

Useful websites

www.bandolier.org.uk/ This is an online evidence-based medicine journal. The glossary, extended essays and learning zone are of great use to students of research.

https://conjointly.com/kb/ The *Research Methods Knowledge Base* is a comprehensive web-based textbook that addresses all the topics in a typical introductory undergraduate or graduate course in social research methods. The section on experimental and quasi-experimental design is quite useful.

www.casp-uk.net The home of the Critical Appraisal Skills Programme and some great tools for checking the quality of research reports.

Chapter 5 Data collection methods and analysis in quantitative research

Chapter aims

After reading this chapter, you will be able to:

- identify the major data collection methods used in quantitative research;
- describe the advantages and disadvantages of the data collection methods used in quantitative research;
- describe the key elements of data analysis in quantitative research;
- demonstrate awareness of the quality issues related to data management in quantitative research.

Introduction

In the previous chapter, quantitative research methodologies were identified as a means of answering questions about cause and effect as well as correlations and associations between variables and as a means of counting both incidence and prevalence. This chapter identifies the main data collection methods used within quantitative research in health and social care and explains how they meet the aims of the chosen methodology. It explores how data are collected and the pros and cons of the approaches, and it examines the use of surveys and questionnaires as data collection methods.

This chapter also looks at data presentation and data analysis in quantitative research and what they serve to demonstrate. It uses examples from the literature and some activities to demonstrate the approach to the reader in a meaningful way. It also illuminates some of the ways in which the process of data presentation and analysis in the quantitative methodologies can be demonstrated to be both valid and reliable.

The aim of this chapter is not to provide an exhaustive account of the data collection methods used in quantitative research nor the accompanying statistics, but rather to present a summary of the main methods used and the reasoning behind the processes and procedures adopted.

Key features

It is clear the quantitative methodologies are concerned with numbers, with understanding associations between variables and with demonstrating cause and effect. Gathering such data requires researchers to engage in much thought not only about what they want to collect but also about how they might collect it and how they might ensure the quality of the process.

The key features of all quantitative study methods are the consistency and accuracy of the data collection process. The consistency (reliability) and accuracy (validity) of the data collection, together with the representativeness of the sample used, ensure that the data collected are suitable to be used to generate findings that can be generalised. Unlike qualitative research, which moves from specific observations towards the generation of more general hypotheses, the purpose of quantitative research is to move from general observations to the generation of more specific outcomes. The specific and well-defined nature of the outcome measures (the research findings) means that the results of quantitative research are often capable of being generalised (that is, applied with a fair degree of certainty outside of the research setting to people and in situations broadly similar to those studied).

Activity 5.1   Reflection

Retrieve your answer to Activity 4.2 and compare what you have discovered about representativeness and generalisability to the concept summary below. Consider why, bearing in mind the explanation given in this chapter, generalisability is so important in establishing the value of evidence used to inform practice.

There is an outline answer at the end of the chapter.

Concept summary: generalisability

Generalisability is an important feature of quantitative research because it allows the researcher to have a fair degree of certainty that the findings of the research apply to people who have the same, or broadly similar, characteristics as the people involved in the study.

Think of it this way: as nurses working in the clinical setting it is important we feel the care we deliver to a patient will work. For example, it is important for us to know the dressing that we apply to a particular wound or the ways in which we prevent the formation of pressure sores are going to be effective. This knowledge is generated by research that has been carried out to demonstrate this. That research has involved people who are broadly similar to the patients we care for, so we have some certainty that the information we apply from the research will be relevant to our patients.

Research into the treatment of post-natal depression applies to people with post-natal depression. The same research will not apply to the treatment of people with depression of a different cause or of a different type, say reactive depression. The research may have taken place in only 100 people with post-natal depression, but it applies to all patients with post-natal depression who are broadly similar to the people who took part in the research. The research is *generalisable* to people with post-natal depression and only those people.

Nurses are familiar with undertaking treatments and care regimes that are broadly similar and work when we apply them time and again to different patients with the same problem. Such regimens are often the product of quantitative research that informs the provision of care, the outcomes of which are broadly speaking predictable. This is the first and most important premise of quantitative study design: it informs practice. As such, it is easy to see how quantitative research might reflect the aspirations of the NMC Standards of Proficiency in Nursing cited at the start of the chapter. These include making evidence-based decisions which are based on an understanding of research practices. It is this very reason, the applicability of research to practice delivery and improvement (evidence-based nursing practice), which prompts registering bodies such as the NMC to place so much emphasis on research, and understanding research, for nursing students (see *Evidence-Based Practice in Nursing*, also in this series; Ellis, 2019).

When discussing the qualitative methodologies, we saw that the researcher is seen as a tool of data collection and that this provides depth and richness to the process. This personal engagement with the collection of data was identified as necessary in enabling the researcher to develop the human interactions that form the basis of qualitative research. We also identified that, because of the interactive nature of the data-collecting methods in qualitative research, these being verbal and observational, it is hard to eradicate bias.

The collection of data within the quantitative methodologies requires researchers to be one step removed from the process, so they remain *objective* and their approach to the process is consistent. This detachment ensures the quality of the data collected is high and there is less room for bias (the introduction of systematic errors) to creep into the data collection process.

The rest of the chapter explores the use of the quantitative data collection methods most commonly used in nursing research: questionnaires, surveys, structured interviews and the collection of clinical (physiological) data. In order to understand the processes involved in the design and delivery of surveys and questionnaires, the principles of how questions are chosen and worded and methods for answering the question selected are explored first. The chapter concludes by examining approaches to data presentation and analysis in quantitative research.

Choosing what questions to ask

The process of choosing what questions to ask within a quantitative research study requires thought, experience, reading of the existing research and reflection. As a guiding principle, the nature of the study and the topic being explored will to some extent predetermine this. When deciding what questions to ask during a study it is important to keep in mind at all times the aims and objectives of the research.

One way in which the researcher can plan the questions to ask during a study is to examine the questions other researchers have used, and successfully (or not) had answered, in similar studies. However, while previous studies in similar areas can provide some general ideas, the exact nature of the research question and the characteristics of the people with whom the research is being undertaken will be important in deciding which questions should be included in any study. For example, if you work in the UK then similar studies undertaken in health systems which are unlike that in the UK, say on the uptake of screening in the USA, where people pay for their care either at the point of use or through insurance, may provide some ideas for the study, but these will need contextualising to the UK situation.

Many quantitative data collection tools already exist. Such tools, usually questionnaires, have been designed to collect defined data from within certain specific groups. Examples of these questionnaires include the Short Form 36 (SF36), which is a 36-question questionnaire that is used in general populations to gain an insight into individuals' perceptions of their own physical and psychological well-being. The SF36 is a useful tool for gaining data about the general well-being of individuals and has been used in many thousands of research projects (**www.sf-36.org**).

Activity 5.2   Reflection

Retrieve your answer to Activity 4.6 and compare it to what you have discovered in the way of pre-validated questionnaires used in quantitative research. Compare what you have found and understand to the examples and explanations within the rest of this chapter.

As the answer is based on your own reflection, there is no outline answer at the end of the chapter.

As well as more general tools, like SF36 and some of those you may have identified in Chapter 4, there are many disease- and function-specific questionnaires in wide use in quantitative research. Disease-specific questionnaires have been especially designed to answer questions about the perceived state of health of individuals with a wide range of diseases. Examples include the Kidney Disease Quality of Life Short Form (KDQOL-SF), used specifically with people with chronic kidney disease, and the MacNew Heart Disease Health-related Quality of Life Instrument (MacNew), which is designed to assess and evaluate the health-related quality of life of people living with heart disease.

As well as questionnaires that apply to people in different health states, there are questionnaires for measuring physical well-being (e.g. the Karnofsky Performance Scale Index), psychological well-being (e.g. the Psychological General Well-being Index), social well-being (e.g. the Social Activities Satisfaction Instrument) and emotional well-being (e.g. the State-Trait Anxiety Index), among others. The benefit of using pre-existing questionnaires comes not only in the time they save, but also in the fact that (if matched appropriately) they often have a high degree of validity and reliability within the populations in which they have been tested.

There is little point in designing questions for quantitative research when existing tools can address the study aims adequately. One note of caution should be given, however: just because a data collection instrument has been widely used and has good reliability and validity it does not mean that it will retain those qualities in every group of individuals with whom it is used. For example, a questionnaire that is designed to measure the quality of life in individuals with renal disease may not apply very well to individuals with heart disease. So pre-existing questionnaires can only be used with certainty in people similar to those in whom the questionnaire has been validated.

Perhaps the most important aspect of the process of deciding which questions to ask is deciding which questions do not need to be included. For example, if you are researching the implementation of a pre-operative fasting regime for general surgery, questions about the gender, age and ethnicity of the people answering the questionnaire may not be important. If, however, you are concerned with the understanding of and adherence to pre-operative patient instructions, it may be relevant to the purposes of the study to gain some insight into whether gender, age and ethnicity have an effect on whether people have actually understood, or been able to comply with, the instructions given to them.

Wording questions for research

Questions must make sense to the person being asked them. This may seem obvious. However, a number of issues can arise in the wording of a question that can make it difficult to understand, let alone answer.

The use of words that have multiple or vague meanings can make a question difficult to answer. For example, when exploring the effects of back pain on individuals, a question such as 'Since you have had your back pain have you been able to go out a lot?' has multiple potential meanings:

- 'go out' may be taken to mean 'go out socially', 'go out shopping' or 'go out into the garden';
- 'a lot' may mean daily, weekly or monthly depending on what is normal for the individual.

Such questions also ignore what the person was able to do before they had back pain and what, therefore, is normal for that individual. It may be more appropriate to ask whether the person's level of activity has changed as a result of the back pain rather than pitching what is clearly an ambiguous question.

Using technical words or jargon in a questionnaire that is to be applied to the general public can mean that the questions are not understood. For example, in nursing we might use terms such as 'venepuncture' or 'taking bloods' to describe the process of taking a blood sample from a patient for subsequent analysis. These terms, while they may have a distinct and clear meaning to us, may confuse or potentially even frighten a lay person. Using technical language in a questionnaire applied to non-professionals assumes that they use the language in the same way that you do.

Activity 5.3   Critical thinking

When you next take a handover, make a note of all of the abbreviations and technical language used. Consider how they might sound to a patient or a new student nurse.

As the answer is based on your own area of practice, there is no outline answer at the end of the chapter.

Avoiding asking more than one question within a question is also important. For example, a question with a yes/no answer such as 'Did you have any pain and nausea following your operation?' may gain a positive response in three situations: the respondent had pain but no nausea; the respondent had nausea but no pain; and the respondent had both pain and nausea. Conversely, the absence of either one of the symptoms might get a negative response when in fact this is not true. Asking a question with a double meaning such as this and getting an inaccurate response means that the validity of the question is poor. That is to say, the question is not actually measuring what it sets out to measure.

As a general rule, therefore, questions should be short and precise, and refer to only one issue of interest.

The use of leading questions can also seriously affect the validity of a study. Leading questions are ones that seem to imply a specific response (see Activity 3.2). Such responses may not truly represent the feelings of the respondents, and this will result in the introduction of bias into the study. This bias means that no confidence can be placed in the answer to a given question, and the question will have to be discarded. Leading questions can easily introduce the Hawthorne effect into a study, that is, where people answer questions in the way in which they think the researcher wants them to (see Chapter 3).

Leading questions are of most concern when they are contained within studies that are evaluative. For example, if you are using a questionnaire to evaluate the use of patient-controlled analgesia (PCA), a question such as 'Do you think the fact that you managed your own pain control was better for you than having to wait for a nurse to bring an injection?' tends to point to two distinct reasons why the individual would be happier with PCA. The first is the phrase 'the fact that you managed'. This places the control of the pain firmly with the individual, who is then responsible if it does not work. The second reason is that it is made quite plain the patient would have had to wait for pain relief if they had not been on PCA. That would not be a good thing, would it?

Open and closed questions

Essentially, there are two distinct types of questions that can be contained within any study: open questions and closed questions. The choice of style of question to be used will depend on how much detail is required in the answers, the overall aim of the study and the background research that has gone into designing the study.

Open questions ask the respondent for knowledge, attitudes or feelings (as one might want to do with a qualitative study, for example). They often begin with 'what', 'why' or 'how'. 'Tell me' or 'describe' may also be used to start open questions. Examples include:

- What is it like to survive cancer?
- Why did you choose to be treated here?
- How was your stay in hospital?
- Tell me what happened when you received your diagnosis.
- Describe the clinic visit in more detail.

Open questions are problematic in quantitative research because they gain any number and variety of answers. The data obtained from these answers tend to contain more depth – assuming people can be bothered to answer them – and they allow the respondents to raise issues important to them. That is the opposite of what we stated the purpose of quantitative research to be at the start of the chapter, which was 'to move from general observations to the generation of more specific outcomes'. The variety and depth of the responses do mean, however, that it is almost impossible for researchers to quantify them in any meaningful way. The pros and cons of open questions are summarised in Table 5.1.

Pros	Cons
Provide rich in-depth data	Difficult to capture all answers
Do not restrict participants' answers	More difficult for participants to answer
Get more detailed answers	More difficult to categorise and analyse answers
Gain good insight into participants' opinions	May produce answers not relevant to the question
Let respondents raise issues	May allow people not to bother to answer questions fully

Table 5.1   Pros and cons of open questions

Closed questions are the exact opposite of open questions and are designed to get either a one-word answer or a very short factual answer – they move us from the general to the more specific. They are very useful for quantitative data collection as the responses given are easily counted and analysed. They are quick and easy for respondents to answer. Because closed questions are quite focused, they tend towards directing people's answers. Examples include:

- Do you feel lucky to have survived cancer?
- Did you choose to be treated here because of our reputation?
- Was your stay in hospital satisfactory?
- Did you understand what you were told when you received your diagnosis?
- Was your clinic visit OK?

Closed questions will often start with words such as: can, did, do, will, was and have.

The pros and cons of closed questions are summarised in Table 5.2.

Pros	Cons
Quick to answer	Can be leading
Easy to understand	Respondents can only answer in ways the question allows
Engage people, including those with limited literacy skills	Respondents cannot raise new issues
Easy to quantify responses	Misinterpretation of the question will not be noticed by the researcher
Avoid overly lengthy answers	The answers are often oversimplified

Table 5.2   Pros and cons of closed questions

Because closed questions are designed to gain short responses, there are sometimes issues with their ability to capture fully the response that an individual wishes to give. This may mean that the findings of a quantitative study have limited validity because the answers gained are less than a true reflection of what the individual respondents wanted to say. They actually capture the answer the respondent is allowed to give in view of the options available to them (see scaling questions especially). This lack of **sensitivity** may be overcome by adapting the way in which closed questions can be responded to.

Scaling question responses

Scaling, or ranking, allows people involved in a study to choose an answer to a question that is closest in meaning to the answer they want to give. Such scales usually take one of three forms in quantitative studies: *agreement, evaluation* or *frequency*.

It is usual for such scales to contain between four and seven options, with five being the most common. These methods of grouping responses are referred to as Likert items in some textbooks.

Agreement scales (Figure 5.1) allow respondents to match their level of agreement with a statement contained within a question. While agreement with the answers available may not be absolute, it is generally sufficient, within the context of the quantitative study, that respondents are invited to choose the response that most closely fits what they think or feel.

Strongly agree	Agree	Undecided	Disagree	Strongly disagree

Figure 5.1   An example of an agreement scale

Evaluation scales (Figure 5.2) allow respondents to answer in a manner that measures how good or bad they rate an experience, process or product. Because of the way they are worded, evaluation scales may encourage respondents to answer questions in a more honest way than an agreement scale, the questions of which can appear to be directive (leading).

Excellent	Very good	Undecided	Poor	Very poor

Figure 5.2   An example of an evaluation scale

Frequency scales (Figure 5.3) allow respondents to choose a response to a question that allows some idea as to whether the response represents their experience on all, some or only a very few occasions.

Always	Usually	Sometimes	Rarely	Never

Figure 5.3   An example of a frequency scale

What can be seen from the three examples is that they invite a response to three slightly different questions: the first seeks agreement with a statement of fact; the second asks the respondent to rate an experience; and the third allows some feedback about whether the quality of an experience is consistently good.

Because each form of scaling gains a slightly different response, it is important the researcher takes care during the design of the questions to refer back to the purpose of the study on a regular basis in order to maintain focus. In some instances it may be appropriate to have a mix of question styles in order to gain a more complete picture of the answers the participants want to give.

Notably, two of the scales presented here allow for a neutral answer (e.g. undecided). This is common in many scales and is generally good practice, although not necessarily the right option in all circumstances (Chyung et al., 2017).

Visual analogue scales

A visual analogue scale (VAS) (Figure 5.4) provides another way of measuring responses to closed questions in a manner that increases their sensitivity. A VAS attempts to measure an attitude or feeling that spans a continuum of values and cannot easily be categorised. In the clinical setting, the use of a VAS may help in understanding the amount of pain a patient is suffering. Pain may range across a continuum from no pain through to severe pain, and the range in a VAS is continuous to reflect this. Pain does not take discrete leaps as the use of an agreement, evaluation or frequency scale might seem to suggest. A VAS is another example of a Likert scale.

| Excellent | → | Very poor |

Figure 5.4   An example of a visual analogue scale

The advantages of the VAS include engaging people with limited literacy skills and in applying measures to variables that are difficult to apply discrete categories to, and this makes the VAS a useful research tool.

By convention, the line used in a VAS is 10 cm long. Because of their highly subjective nature, VASs are not easy to use to compare the scores given between individuals, but they have great benefits when trying to quantify the changes in a feeling or symptom – for example the amount of pain an individual feels. These scales have the disadvantage that the response needs to be physically measured, for example with a ruler, in order to be quantifiable, so more time is needed to collect the data.

In children, or adults with very limited literacy skills, the use of pictures instead of a written-on single-line scale can enhance the ability of the researcher to collect data. Perhaps the best example is the use of the 'faces pain scale' which rates the pain that a child is feeling by relating it to the emotion displayed on cartoon faces (Spagrud et al., 2003) (e.g. see **www.wongbakerfaces.org**).

Activity 5.4   Research and finding out

When you are next in the practice setting, take the time to look at the various tools you use to measure signs and symptoms in patients. Examples might include a pain scale, a symptom and concern checklist or self-reported psychiatric symptoms. What is important for you to realise, as you reflect on these, is that nurses are already familiar with the collection of quantitative data in their daily clinical practice.

As the answer is based on your own area of practice, there is no outline answer at the end of the chapter.

Surveys

Key features

Cross-sectional surveys attempt to quantify the prevalence (the amount) of a variable (e.g. feeling, attitude or opinion) in a group of individuals at a given point in time. These surveys set out to be either descriptive or correlational. A descriptive study only presents single variables as the amount in which they occur within the study sample (e.g. the number of people with COVID-19), while a correlational study looks for associations between two or more variables (e.g. whether age correlates with satisfaction with hospital care).

While a cross-sectional survey may be able to demonstrate an apparent correlation between two variables, as it is not longitudinal (it does not carry through time), as it is not a method that can explore a cause-and-effect relationship; that is, it shows no temporal sequence. (To remind yourself about this distinction, see Chapter 4.)

Some surveys take place at more than one given point in time, for example:

- a survey which takes place over a period of time, e.g. a new patient satisfaction survey undertaken over a six-month period;
- more than one separate, but connected, surveys, e.g. patient satisfaction surveys for visit 1, 2, 3, etc., to a specific clinic;
- a cohort study using longitudinal survey methods (Lynn, 2021).

Broadly speaking, surveys can be undertaken prospectively (that is, in real time), retrospectively (that is, using previously collected data) or using a mixture of both approaches.

Prospective surveys

Prospective surveys are undertaken to ascertain the feelings, thoughts and attitudes of people about a service or product at the point at which they receive the service or use the product. This has the advantage that the data collected can all be standardised, ensuring their reliability. That is, the ways in which the data are collected are managed by the researcher.

Prospective data collection has the added advantage that it does not require individuals to have to remember a previous event; they can record feelings in real time. This means that recall bias is eliminated from the study; it can, however, mean answers are raw and lack the finesse of answers which may have been reflected on.

Retrospective surveys

Retrospective surveys are studies that collect data about past events. Some surveys may use previously collected data – for example, routinely recorded data on outpatient waiting times – or they may collect data from individuals about a service or product that they experienced in the past.

In common with all retrospective studies, retrospective surveys are prone to issues that relate to the ability of an individual to recall past events (recall bias); clearly, time can change a person's perceptions and memories of an event. Retrospective surveys using previously collected data are also subject to the quality of the data collection processes at the time. There may be issues with reliability (especially inter-rater), and validity, because data were not collected according to a standardised format and the consistency of the data may be questionable. That said, retrospective surveys which rely on recall allow the respondent to have reflected on an experience and the answers gained may therefore be better thought through.

Concept summary: recall bias

Recall bias can prove a major obstacle in the execution of any study. It arises in a number of ways, all of which are systematic. People who had a bad experience of care may be more likely to remember it as being bad than people who had a reasonable experience, who may, with the passing of time, subsequently remember the experience as being good. Known examples of this phenomenon include mothers of children with birth defects, who are more likely to recall the use of alcohol and smoking during pregnancy than mothers whose children are born healthy, and people with lung cancer who relate a more accurate smoking history than people who do not have lung cancer.

The quality and consistency of data collection and recording outside a research project are variable. For example, the notes recorded by two triage nurses working in the same emergency department may be quite different, even if they are seeing people with similar conditions. This is a result of normal human variation, but it means the collection of data for research purposes may be incomplete. Even within research there need to be safeguards in place, especially where more than one person is collecting data, to make sure there is some consistency (inter-rater reliability).

Activity 5.5   Research and finding out

In order to understand recall bias, try to remember everything you have eaten or drunk for the last week and write it all down. After you have done this keep a food and drink diary for a week. Compare the two lists after the second week and see if your recalled list appears as complete as the one you made prospectively. Reflect on why this might be.

As the answer is based on your own findings, there is no outline answer at the end of the chapter.

Advantages

Surveys have the advantage of being quick and easy to do, making them relatively cheap. Because surveys are so commonplace in society they are easily understood by people, and therefore generally quite user-friendly.

Surveys can be undertaken using a variety of different approaches, which usually means the use of questionnaires (which may be postal or administered via face-to-face interviews, telephone interviews, e-mail, online chat rooms, via social media or dedicated websites). The variety of techniques available means that there has to be a degree of thought applied to how a survey is to be undertaken, with some topic areas more suitable for a particular method than others – for example, it may be less appropriate to use social media to survey older people's satisfaction with healthcare provision than it is younger people's, while some young people might not be as truthful face to face as some more mature participants.

On the whole, face-to-face interviews yield the fullest responses with the highest uptake of respondents. This is because it is harder to refuse a face-to-face interview than it is to ignore an e-mail and because there is the opportunity in a face-to-face interview for the questioner to clarify any questions the respondent does not understand, as well as to clarify responses.

Disadvantages

Because of their speed and the fact they need to be user-friendly, surveys tend to be superficial. Furthermore, the quality of the data collected in a survey is limited by the willingness and ability of the individuals included in the study to answer (truthfully) the questions posed to them. The willingness of participants to answer the questions is related to the topic of the research, the questions that are being asked and how the questions are being asked.

When not filled in face to face, surveys may be responded to by people other than those they were sent to – this can potentially bias the study as it affects the sample selection. Mailed and e-mailed surveys are easily ignored and, if they can be returned anonymously, it is hard to chase up recipients.

People who respond to surveys are self-selecting, that is, they choose to take part. This self-selection may result in bias, with individuals with a very good or very bad experience being more likely to take part, for instance, than people having an average or normal experience. This will affect representativeness and therefore generalisability.

Structured interviews

Structured interviews are interviews in which the questions to be asked and the order in which they are to be asked are decided before the interview takes place. The interviewer has a list of the questions to ask and then asks them. There is no room allowed for deviation from the interview script, which has to be delivered in the same order using the same words on each occasion it is used (Tod, 2015).

Structured interviews have the advantage that all of the interviewees are questioned in the same way, following the same protocol. This makes the job of the interviewer that little bit easier. It allows there to be some consistency (reliability) within a research process that involves one researcher but also in studies that involve more than one person in the data collection; in the latter case it increases inter-rater reliability.

Concept summary: structured interviews

Structured interviews are in some respects similar to the documents used when undertaking an assessment of a patient on admission to a ward. It is important that all of the same data are collected in the same manner so that everyone who is later involved in the patient's care has access to the data in a structured and consistent manner. Deviating from the assessment process, neglecting to collect some pieces of information or failing to include all of the usual documentation in the assessment leads to confusion and the potential for something important to be missed. Within the structured interview protocol, failure to gather data in the same way on each occasion means the data will not easily be compared and that there is confusion about what questions the research has actually answered, impacting both the validity and reliability of the research.

It is easier when writing up a study involving structured interviews to include in the research paper the list of questions asked and the order in which they were asked. This has the advantage of making it clear to readers exactly what was asked, so they can then compare this to the answers given and decide for themselves if the findings of the study, as presented by the researcher, appear reasonable, and indeed whether the questions used actually address the aims and purpose of the study.

The main disadvantage of structured interviews is that they tend to gain less full responses from the interviewees, as the answers they can give are constrained by the type and nature of the questions asked. Structured interviews are sometimes used as a method of data collection in quantitative research where there is a requirement for all of the data to be collected in the same way using the same questions in order to maintain the consistency (reliability) of the data collection.

Questionnaires

As a method of data collection, questionnaires are everywhere. There are many different styles of questionnaire, each designed to do a different job. Some questionnaires are specially written for an individual piece of research, while others have been designed to be used repeatedly to measure variables within defined populations – pre-validated questionnaires. Dowrick et al. (2015) point out that a failure to use a validated questionnaire for a specified population can lead to measurement errors which might invalidated a study's findings.

Questionnaires can be delivered in a number of ways, which include face to face, via post, via e-mail and online via website or, increasingly, on social media platforms.

There are advantages and disadvantages to all of the different types and delivery methods. The nature of the research and the research question itself guide the exact choice of how a questionnaire is both designed and delivered. There are few hard-and-fast rules about what a good questionnaire should contain in the way of questions or ways of answering. Nor are there any guiding principles that allow researchers to know which method of delivering the questionnaire is most appropriate for the research question they are investigating.

What is important in the choice of style of questions and mode of delivery of the questionnaire is that the researcher has thought about the potential pros and cons, given the nature of the research question and the people to whom the questionnaire is to be applied. The best researchers will refer, as we have seen in Chapter 1, to the existing literature in the topic area and use the lessons learnt from this to guide their decisions. For the novice researcher this is particularly important, as is the engagement of the help of a more experienced researcher and, potentially, a statistician who can advise on question designs that will support the subsequent process of data analysis.

Key features

For the quantitative questionnaire, the thing that is most important is that the answers collected are a true reflection of the question asked, that is, that the questions are valid. This may seem obvious. However, writing a question in such a way that it will be understood to mean the same thing by all the people who will read it is not easy.

The second most important aspect of questionnaire design is to ensure that responses are gained from as many of the target sample as possible. This means thought needs to go into not only the questions asked but also where, when and how the questioning is to take place. In a student or young population, a questionnaire may work well when placed in an online environment, but the opposite may be true for older people or those on low incomes who may not have access to, or be used to using, the internet (although this is increasingly not the case).

Questionnaires often need to elicit more than one type of data. The main data relate to the topic of interest while other data are needed to record the demographic and other characteristics of respondents, which may be used to identify correlations or trends. The length of any questionnaire should be limited to gaining the data needed for the study and no more. It is often wise to include some filtering questions at the start so that people not eligible for the study are identified early on and so do not proceed to answer the whole questionnaire – this is particularly common and useful in online surveys.

Generally, it is a good idea to phrase questions positively rather than negatively, for example, using 'Was your pain well managed after surgery?' as opposed to 'Was your pain poorly controlled after surgery?' Negative questioning can, however, be used to check two things. First, when asking for an opinion about something, asking the same question later on in the questionnaire but in the opposite way can be used to check the **internal consistency** of respondents' answers – so if they answer 'disagree' to the ranking of a positive question, they should answer 'agree' to the ranking of a nega-tive question. Second, it is possible to see if the respondent is actually reading all of the questions rather than assuming their content. If they are assuming the content and the question format varies, this is likely to result in a few questions to which the answers do not correspond. As a general rule, if the respondents' answers are more than 70 per cent consistent, the survey is considered to be acceptable.

Other ways of checking the quality of the questioning process include the use of open questions that allow respondents to record their own response and comparing these to the closed responses. Repeated measures designs allow the researcher to apply the questionnaire to the same person at different points in time to see if there is consist-ency. Of course, this type of design is onerous and relies on a respondent being willing to fill out the same questionnaire twice. The disadvantage of this approach arises when the research relates to thoughts, feelings and opinions that are subject to change over time anyway.

There are a number of routes to checking the quality of a questionnaire being used for the first time. Using experts in the topic being studied to help write the questions can be fruitful as they often know the sorts of ideas and misconceptions people have. Doing a pilot study of the questionnaire using the sort of people who will be involved in the main study is also a useful way of ensuring the questions make sense and filling in the questionnaire is not too onerous.

The length of a questionnaire will impact on the response rates achieved. A shorter tick-box questionnaire will always gain more responses than long, more complex ones. It would be wrong to think that a long questionnaire is necessarily of better quality than a short one that is better focused, and equally it would be wrong to use a short tick-box questionnaire when the answers sought are complex or in-depth.

The order in which questions appear has an impact on whether or not people decide to fill in a questionnaire, as do the quality and nature of the questioning involved. Once people have committed some time to filling in a questionnaire, they are more likely to finish it. The general rules for sequencing questions are summa-rised below.

Concept summary: rules about sequencing questions

- go from general to specific;
- go from easy to harder;
- go from factual to more abstract;
- start with closed-format questions (scaled);
- start with questions about the main subject;
- don't start with personal or demographic questions.

Administering questionnaires

There are many ways of administering a questionnaire. The choice of delivery will tend to be driven by the nature of the questions and the sample being questioned. Self-administered questionnaires may be posted in the mail, placed online (e.g. in a topical chat room), e-mailed or left in a pertinent clinical area. Interviewer-administered questionnaires may be undertaken face to face, over the telephone or, increasingly, via the internet.

There are a number of pros and cons to each approach, and these need to be considered before launching into the questioning process. Table 5.3 summarises the pros of each approach.

	Self-administered questionnaires	Interviewer-administered questionnaires
Pros	Quick, cheap, easy to administer; convenient for respondent; confidentiality and anonymity easily preserved; easily standardised format and limited researcher input needed. Respondent can choose when to do the questionnaire. Good for embarrassing topics. If done electronically can go direct into analysing database	Interviewer can clarify questions; allows participation by people who are illiterate; virtually guarantees a high response rate; quality and completeness of questionnaires may be higher. Can select the participants
Cons	The potential respondent may choose not to do the questionnaire, so response rate may be low. The respondent may not understand some questions. Cannot gauge truthfulness of responses; cannot ensure all questions are answered. Impersonal. Respondents are self-selecting and may not be representative of the population of interest	Interviewer may influence the responses. Time consuming and expensive. Not good for potentially embarrassing subjects. Gaining access to people can be problematic

Table 5.3 Pros and cons of self- and interviewer-administered questionnaires

Presenting and analysing quantitative data

By their very nature quantitative studies produce outputs – findings – that are quantifiable. This means the outputs of a quantitative study include data that use numbers. The presentation of data from a quantitative study includes data that describe both the characteristics of the participants and the findings of the study. As well as the descriptive data, statistics may be presented that make inferences about what the study has found. These two types of statistical data are called **descriptive statistics** and **inferential statistics**.

Essentially, descriptive statistics describe only the range, measures of central tendency, frequency and distribution of certain characteristics within the study. Inferential statistics, on the other hand, present data about the **probabilities** associated with the outcomes of the study. The following sections discuss in limited detail the sort of data that should be included in the report of a quantitative research study and why. Some explanation of how different statistical findings are arrived at is offered. You are encouraged to look in the specialist texts suggested at the end of the chapter if you want to be able to understand any of the information presented here in more detail or if you need to undertake any statistical tests for your own research.

Descriptive statistics

Descriptive statistics do exactly what they say. That is, they describe patterns of data within a dataset. Descriptive statistics are used to give the reader some idea of the make-up of a study, the numbers of people involved, their spread of age, gender, ethnicity and the like. The exact data presented depend on the nature and purpose of the study undertaken.

Descriptive statistics are concerned with the presentation of summaries of the data generated during a study, which may run to thousands of pieces of data. It is for this reason the data are clustered or counted and described rather than all the individual pieces of data presented. Examples of the ways in which descriptive statistics are presented include percentages, basic calculations, graphs, charts and tables. Descriptive statistics present an account of the data, with particular reference to its central tendency, distribution and frequency.

Measures of central tendency

Measures of central tendency give the reader a good idea of some of the central, or average, values of a set of data. There are a number of measures of central tendency, each with particular messages they convey to the reader. They also allow the researcher to make some statements about the nature of the sample from which the data were collected and the overall results of the study.

The arithmetic mean

This is what is commonly known as an **average**. The **mean** is calculated by adding all of the values in a dataset together and then dividing by the number of values. For example, all the ages of the people involved in the study divided by the number of people involved in the study would give us the mean age (Figure 5.5).

Find the arithmetic mean of the data: 7, 5, 4, 6, 7, 14, 11, 5, 9, 10, 12

$7 + 5 + 4 + 6 + 7 + 14 + 11 + 5 + 9 + 10 + 12 = 90$

$90 ÷ 11 = 8.2$

Figure 5.5   An example of how to calculate a mean

The mean uses all the observations in the dataset and each observation affects the mean. It is sensitive to extreme values (i.e. if there are one or two extreme values in a small set of data, they will affect the mean disproportionately). The mean has valuable mathematical properties that make it convenient for use in inferential statistical analysis, as we will see later in the chapter.

As with most simple statistics, the mean can be calculated for large datasets using a simple computerised spreadsheet or statistical package.

The median

The **median** is the middle value in an *ordered* set of values (Figure 5.6). If there is an even number of data in the set, the median is the mean of the two middle numbers. The median provides a better measure of central tendency, on the whole, than the mean when there are some extremely large or small observations in a dataset – this is especially true where the dataset consists of a small number of values.

Find the median of the data: 7, 5, 4, 6, 7, 14, 11, 5, 9, 10, 12

Put the data in order: 4, 5, 5, 6, 7, 7, 9, 10, 11, 12, 14

Select the middle value: 4, 5, 5, 6, 7, 7, 9, 10, 11, 12, 14 = 7

Figure 5.6   An example of how to calculate a median

Unlike the mean, the median does not have important mathematical properties for use in future calculations. The median is often used when quoting survival data in the clinical setting and refers to the point in time to which 50 per cent of patients with a given condition will be expected to survive; for example, median survival for people with breast cancer is now greater than ten years – that is, half of people with breast cancer will survive at least ten years.

The mode

The **mode** is the most frequently occurring number in a set of observations. Some data-sets may have two modes, in which case we say the data are *bimodal* (Figure 5.7). Where a dataset has more than two modes it is referred to as *multimodal.* The mode is not usually a helpful measure of central tendency because there can be more than one mode or even no mode. Like the median, the mode does not have important mathematical properties for future use.

Find the median of the data: 7, 5, 4, 6, 7, 14, 11, 5, 9, 10, 12

The numbers 5 and 7 both appear twice; each other number appears only once.

The dataset is therefore bimodal with the numbers 5 and 7 both being the modes of this dataset.

Figure 5.7   An example of how to calculate a mode

The mode might be useful in reporting people's attitudes or opinions, especially when the data collected are nominal or categorical. What most people think about a clinical service might be helpful in designing service improvement, so mode does have good clinical applications.

The range

The **range** is the difference between the largest and smallest observation of a dataset. Typically, the smallest and largest number – for example the age of the youngest and oldest person in a study, are reported.

The major disadvantage of the range is that it does not include all of the observations. Only the two most extreme values are included, and these two numbers may be untypical observations.

Using the same data as Figure 5.7, therefore, the range of the observations is from 4 to 14 and is therefore 10.

Standard deviation

This is perhaps the most poorly understood of the descriptive statistics reported in any study. Standard deviation is essentially the mean of the difference from the mean of each of the observations being reported. The best way to understand standard deviation is perhaps to see one worked out long-hand (Figure 5.8).

1.	Find the arithmetic mean of the data: 7, 5, 4, 6, 7, 14, 11, 5, 9, 10, 12 = 8.2
2.	Find the difference between each observation and the mean (e.g. 7 – 8.2 = –1.2).
	–1.2, –3.2, –4.2, –2.2, –1.2, 5.8, 2.8, –3.2, 0.8, 1.8, 3.8
3.	Square these differences (for example –1.2 x –1.2 = 1.44) (the square of a negative giving a positive value).
	1.44 + 10.24 + 17.64 + 4.84 + 1.44 + 33.64 + 7.84 + 10.24 + 0.64 + 3.24 + 14.44
4.	Add together these squared differences = 105.64
5.	Divide this number by the number of observations minus one = 9.6.
6.	Find the square root of this number = **3.1**

Figure 5.8 An example of how to calculate a standard deviation

The standard deviation of a set of data that are normally distributed (i.e. data that when graphed show a bell shape) – as is the case in much biological data – enables the reader to get a feel for where most of the variables within a dataset lie. Something in the region of 68 per cent of all the data will lie within one standard deviation of the mean, while 95 per cent of observations will lie within two standard deviations. The reporting of the mean and the standard deviation of a given dataset allows the researcher and subsequent readers of the research to get a good feel for where the centre as well as where most of the values within the dataset lie.

It is a great relief to know that it is usually not necessary for the researcher to have to calculate these descriptive statistics manually as all spreadsheet and statistical programs have this facility.

Activity 5.6   Research and finding out

Collect together the heights and weights of a few of your classmates or the people in your house. Using the definitions and examples above, calculate the mean, median, mode, standard deviation and range of this data. You might like to do this long-hand and then check your answers using a spreadsheet program.

As the answer is based on your own data, there is no outline answer at the end of the chapter.

Inferential statistics

Descriptive statistics are used to reduce down a dataset of numbers into a few uncomplicated values that are represented either as numbers or in graphs. In this sense, descriptive statistics are like a book summary – they get across the basic idea without the detail.

The purpose of inferential statistics within the research process is to demonstrate that the findings of the research extend beyond the sample within which the research was carried out. Extending beyond the study sample to the population from which the sample was drawn requires that inferential statistics go beyond the data available as a result of the study. Because inferential statistics go beyond the actual data available via the study, they are invariably subject to error. Because of this potential for error the term inferential statistics and not deductive statistics is used – that is, the statistics infer (suggest) rather than absolutely prove something.

Concept summary: inferential statistics

Inferential is a word used to indicate that the statistical findings are subject to some presumption on the part of the person doing the statistics. This presumptiveness is reflected in two ways: first, the findings of the inferential statistics are usually presented as probabilities (p values), which are explained below; second, the findings of all quantitative studies remain open to be proved or disproved by subsequent studies (as was discussed in Chapter 4).

Inferential statistics use a number of processes to make sure that the suppositions are as reasonable as they can be. What this means is, despite the fact the findings are not 100 per cent certain, we can place a fair degree of confidence in the statistical findings of any quantitative research.

The findings of inferential statistics are usually expressed in terms of probability. The probability to which they refer is the likelihood of the findings of the study being found by chance. In other words, probability shows us how much confidence we can have that the findings of the study did not occur by fluke.

Probabilities are expressed as p values. For example, a p value of 0.1 (usually written up as $p = 0.1$) would mean that there is a 10 per cent chance that the findings of the study occurred by chance. Think about how this works: 0.1 is one-tenth of the number 1, while 10 per cent is one-tenth of 100 per cent, so they are essentially the same thing.

Activity 5.7   Research and finding out

If $p = 0.1$ means a 10 per cent chance or 1/10th chance that the findings of the study occurred by chance, try to work out what the following mean:

$p = 0.2$
$p = 0.05$
$p = 0.01$
$p = 0.001$

Express your answers as a percentage and as a non-decimal fraction.

There are answers at the end of the chapter.

In order to understand *p* values better, it is important to understand that the lower the number the better the result. For example, $p = 0.02$ suggests that the findings of the study occurring by chance are four times less than if the result were $p = 0.08$; while $p = 0.05$ suggests that the findings of the study occurring by chance are four times less than if the result were $p = 0.2$.

Sometimes statistics are presented using less than (<) and greater than (>) symbols. Given that the smaller the number, the less chance there is that the result of the study occurred by chance, clearly the best results will generally be small and the < is preferable. So a result of $p < 0.05$ means there is less than a 1 in 20 chance that the results of the study occurred by chance and this is a lower probability than $p = 0.05$.

By convention, if there is no good statistical reason, a result of $p < 0.05$ (probability of less than or equal to (≤) 1 in 20) is accepted as a statistically significant result. Statistically significant means it is accepted that the results of the study did not occur by chance, or that at the very least the chance of them occurring by chance is so small as to be insignificant (Grove and Cipher, 2020). Sometimes in sociological studies a *p* value of < 0.1 is accepted as statistically significant, as the burden of proof in this type of study may be less than that of other quantitative studies.

Statistical significance is different from clinical significance. Some studies that demonstrate a weak statistical finding may well be important, or significant, enough for clinicians to consider adopting the findings. The most important reason for this is the fact that some studies have small sample sizes, which can seriously affect the statistics. Weak statistical significance in small studies tends to suggest that the study might have reached a more statistically significant result had it been bigger, and for many clinical purposes, when taken together with findings from other research, audit and clinical experience, may be enough on which to base a tentative change (Ellis, 2019). Situations when this might be especially important include those where the study involves a rare condition, making the likelihood of getting together a large sample for the study itself small.

Before looking briefly at some of the inferential statistical tests that can be used in analysing quantitative research data, it is perhaps worth understanding the different types of data that can be analysed.

Data types

During the collection of data for any study there are a number of ways in which the data can be categorised (Table 5.4). Categorising the data helps in the selection of both the descriptive and the inferential statistics to be applied to the data and is something that should be thought about and designed into the study at the start, in order to ensure that the correct data are collected in the correct manner to allow later presentation or analysis.

Data type	Type of measurement	Example
Categorical	Nominal (has no inherent order)	Diagnosis; ethnicity
	Ordinal (categories with an order)	Likert scale; self-reported health status
	Binary (a form of ordinal involving only two groups)	Gender; illness or wellness
Quantitative (interval or ratio) (units of measurement applied as a rule)	Discrete (as a rule these are whole numbers)	Number of patients on a ward; blood group
	Continuous (can take any value, but usually measured, counted or ordered to a predetermined degree of accuracy)	Height; weight; temperature

Table 5.4 Types of quantitative data

Different data types can be presented in different ways using descriptive statistics. Table 5.5 shows the measures of central tendency (types of average) that can be used to describe different data types.

	Type of average		
	Mean	**Median**	**Mode**
Nominal			X
Ordinal		X	X
Interval/ratio	X	X	X

Table 5.5 Measures of central tendency that can be used with specific quantitative data types

Parametric/non-parametric data

Before applying any inferential statistics to a dataset it is important to ascertain whether the data need to be analysed using parametric or non-parametric statistical tests. Parametric data are data that when plotted on a histogram present a bell-shaped curve. Such data are said to be normally distributed (Petrie and Sabin, 2020). Normal distribution is most often achieved in datasets that are large and that contain naturally occurring measurements (such as heights of a group).

Data that are normally distributed have at their peak the mean of the data with about 68 per cent of the data values lying within one standard deviation of the mean, 95 per cent within two and 99.7 per cent within three (Figure 5.9). As well as plotting the distribution curve, there are statistical tests that can be applied to data to see if they are normally distributed and therefore whether parametric tests can be used in the analysis of the data.

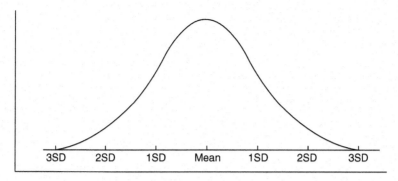

Figure 5.9 The normal distribution curve

Parametric tests tend to be the preferred form of statistical testing because they produce more powerful results on the whole. However, the incorrect use of parametric tests in small datasets, or with data that are not normally distributed, can lead to misleading results.

The exact choice of test to be used with different forms of data is a matter of careful consideration that is best decided before data for a study are collected, and in conjunction with a statistician. Given the variety and number of statistical tests available, it is beyond the scope of this book to present them here. Instead we will consider the use and interpretation of two commonly used statistical tests that will allow us to get some insight into how inferential statistics work.

The *t*-test

The first common inferential statistic is the *t*-test. The *t*-test is used to gauge whether the means of two groups are statistically different from each other. Not only this, the *t*-test is sensitive to the spread of the individual results within each group (as represented by the standard deviation; see page 128) and the number of observations in each set of data.

The *t*-test comes in two forms: the standard *t*-test compares the means from two separate (independent) groups (as one might find in a randomised controlled trial, where there is an experimental group and a control group) and the paired *t*-test measures before-and-after measurements in the same individual (where an intervention has applied, for example) or in two paired (or matched, such as for gender, age and ethnicity) individuals.

The standard *t*-test can only be applied to data that are continuous (Table 5.4) and follow the normal distribution (Figure 5.9) and where the two groups' standard deviations (Figure 5.8) are broadly similar.

Case study

In her RCT into the effects of using unfolding case studies as opposed to traditional case studies and the development of critical thinking skills in student nurses, Englund (2020) compared exam scores attained by the students taught by each methodology. Using the standard *t*-test, she showed that the mean exam scores were significantly higher for the intervention group (unfolding case studies) as opposed to the control group (standard case studies). The *t*-test value, 299, gives a $p < 0.001$. This means that the likelihood of the outcome occurring by chance was less than (<) 0.1 per cent or one in one thousand.

The paired *t*-test has slightly different rules in that they apply to the set of difference scores; the observations should be normally distributed (for both readings); the readings should be paired and in preference the dependent variable will be measured on an interval or ratio scale.

Three applications of the paired *t*-test that are useful but slightly different are: to compare the efficacy of two forms of eye drops for hay fever relief when drop A is applied to the right eye and drop B to the left eye in the same individual (this gives a binary result (relief or no relief)) where individuals are their own 'pair'; to measure the impact of an exercise regime over a one-month period in people weighed at the start and the end of the exercise programme (continuous data) where again individuals are their own pair; and to measure the growth rate in twins where one is given a supplement and the other a normal diet (here the pairing is closely matched).

It is worth understanding here that the statistical formulation of the *t*-test takes into account the means and standard deviations of the measured value as well as the numbers of individuals enrolled in each arm of the study. Because of this, *t*-tests are greatly affected by the numbers of people in a study and the size of whatever effect the study is measuring.

The chi-square test

The other important statistical test widely used in quantitative research is the *chi-square* (χ^2) *test*. The chi-square test can be applied to data that report frequency (categorical data), and are of an adequate size, and where the categories being used are mutually exclusive (that is, no one subject can be in any two groups at the same time). The chi-square test basically allows us to see if the distributions (counts) of categorical data differ between one or more groups. It is worth noting that the chi-square test can only be used on actual numbers and not percentages, proportions or means.

Case study

In their cross-sectional study examining the factors influencing the knowledge and skills of nurses acting in a triage capacity in Ethiopia, Duko et al. (2019) found working experience ($p < 0.05$) and triage experience ($p < 0.05$) were the factors most clearly associated with the nurses skills at triage. This suggests there is a less than one in 20 (5 per cent) probability that these findings were due to chance.

Activity 5.8   Research and finding out

Go online and find the two studies mentioned above (you may find it useful to do this via your NHS or university ATHENS account). Once you have found the papers look at the way in which the data are presented and compare this to what you have learnt about data in this chapter. Once you have done this, find a few other research papers and compare how they present their research statistics (both descriptive and inferential) to what you have learnt in this chapter.

As the answer is based on your own research, there is no outline answer at the end of the chapter.

Chapter summary

This chapter has introduced you to the key methods used in data collection in the types of quantitative research that nurses most frequently undertake, that is, questionnaires and surveys. Such methods are often used to answer questions about the perceptions and attitudes of participants to the care they have received.

We have established that the validity and reliability of the data collected are affected by the ways in which questions are worded and presented. Validity, which is about ensuring that a research tool measures what it sets out to measure, is affected by the choice of questions used, while reliability is ensured when the data have been collected in a way that is readily reproducible.

We have seen that there are a variety of ways that both surveys and questionnaires can be undertaken and that the choice of approach is affected by the type of question being asked. Sometimes the nature of the questions asked requires sensitive face-to-face delivery, while on other occasions the sheer volume that can be achieved by a self-completion questionnaire enables a study to attain a high degree of statistical significance.

(Continued)

(Continued)

We have seen how to present and analyse the data from a quantitative study and that decisions about how to analyse and present data need to be made before data collection has started. We have seen that numerical data can be dealt with in two ways: descriptive statistics – which merely describes the data – and inferential statistics – which makes inferences about the data that go beyond the data collected. Making inferences about the data that go beyond the sample means that the findings of the study become more generalisable, with the likelihood of the finding being a result of chance being represented by the p value calculated.

Activities: brief outline answers

Activity 5.1   Reflection (page 109)

You should notice that your definition and the definition given identify how the sample used in a study needs to be similar to the sample to which the study's findings will be applied to ensure that there are no variables, known or unknown, that would affect the study's findings.

Activity 5.7   Research and finding out (page 130)

$p = 0.2$ means 20 per cent or 1/5th chance

$p = 0.05$ means 5 per cent or 1/20th chance

$p = 0.01$ means 1 per cent or 1/100th chance

$p = 0.001$ means 0.1 per cent or 1/1000th chance

Further reading

Ellis, P (2019) *Evidence-Based Practice in Nursing* (4th edn). London: Sage.

Especially Chapter 1, which discusses where evidence for practice might come from.

Plichta, SB and Kelvin, E (eds) (2013) *Munro's Statistical Methods for Health Care Research* (6th edn). London: Wolters Kluwer/Lippincott Williams and Wilkins.

A very clear and comprehensive book covering major statistical methods.

Polit, DF and Beck, CT (2020) *Nursing Research: Generating and Assessing Evidence for Nursing Practice* (11th edn). London: Wolters Kluwer/Lippincott Williams & Wilkins.

Particularly Part 3, 'Designing and conducting quantitative studies to generate evidence for nursing'.

Useful websites

http://mste.illinois.edu/hill/dstat/dstat.html A rather wacky but informative introduction to descriptive statistics.

www.england.nhs.uk/wp-content/uploads/2018/01/bitesize-guide-writing-an-effective-questionnaire.pdf NHS England on how to write an effective questionnaire to gain insight into patient experiences.

https://conjointly.com/kb/descriptive-statistics/ A concise but useful introduction to descriptive statistics.

https://conjointly.com/kb/research-data-analysis/ Some very useful information about descriptive and inferential statistics.

https://conjointly.com/kb/inferential-statistics/ A very helpful guide to inferential statistics.

www.wongbakerfaces.org One example of a visual analogue 'faces pain scale'.

Chapter 6 Multiple methods, evaluation and action research

Chapter aims

After reading this chapter, you will be able to:

- identify the main evaluative research methodologies used in health and social care;
- describe the type of research questions the different research methodologies can be used to answer;
- demonstrate awareness of how samples are chosen for evaluative studies;
- briefly describe the key methods of data collection used in each methodology and how these augment each other in the evaluation process.

Introduction

So far in this book we have seen that research methodologies are split between those that sit within the qualitative and those that sit within the quantitative paradigm (world view). We have explored some of the methods used within these methodologies and noted how the findings of these types of research might be analysed. In this chapter we will explore the idea that some approaches to research sit within both paradigms and use more than one methodology and/or a mix of methods in order to answer questions which have a bearing on practice.

It is important at this stage to recognise that research in nursing (and in health and social care in general) should seek to change practice for the better. Nursing is all about action – that is, doing things for, and perhaps more importantly *with*, patients, their families and carers in order to improve their lives. It is beyond the scope of this book to explore this idea in any detail, but the concepts of using evidence – of which research is only one element – to inform and improve nursing practice are explored in some detail in *Evidence-Based Practice in Nursing*, also in this series (Ellis, 2019).

In this chapter, we examine the concepts underpinning the use of triangulated research methodologies and methods, evaluation research, action research and rapid appraisals. The purpose of this exploration is to broaden the understanding of approaches to research in health and social care, and, importantly, what they can be used to achieve.

The key feature of the research approaches discussed in this chapter is their focus on the practice of nursing and not on the generation of ideas for later application. That is, the processes involved in evaluation and action research are focused on solving clinical and practice issues in *real time*. In this respect they differ greatly from the methodologies described elsewhere in the book, which have focused on the generation of knowledge leading to the need for further research and/or the need for the generation of strategies and policies for the adoption of the findings of the research into clinical practice.

The use of a single methodology in research has been described as *methodological separatism* (Matta, 2019). Methodological separatism arises out of the fact that various researchers within different disciplines believe the human world can only be studied in ways that are distinct and separate from the non-human world. For example, we can study the healing of a broken bone using radiographic and scientific techniques (non-human), but to understand what it is like to experience the healing of a broken bone it is necessary to ask someone who has experienced first-hand what it is like (human). It is not a debate so much about whether qualitative or quantitative research is more legitimate or better. Rather, this separatist view of the world regards humanity and the study of humanity as being something completely separate from everything else.

This separatist view is perhaps too simplistic for the meaningful study of humans, healthcare and nursing in that it fails to recognise the interconnectedness of human biology, sociology, psychology, politics, spirituality and philosophy. We are all aware, as nurses, that the activities of daily living are interconnected. The biological reality of pain affects the psychological well-being of patients. Psychological distress impacts on their social well-being. Their social well-being impacts on the way in which they view the world. The way in which they view the world impacts on the way in which they experience pain, and so the cycle goes on.

Research in nursing involves research into people, and methodological separatism fails to recognise the complexity of human beings and the ways in which our social and biological beings are inextricably linked.

The use of **triangulation** of research methodologies and methods is intended to demonstrate that healthcare problems are complex and the solutions to them are therefore complex and multifaceted. That is to say, high-quality healthcare, and nursing care in particular, is about more than the mere management or curing of disease and as much about the experience of the care from the point of view of the patient. To this end, the triangulation of research methods allows the exploration of both the quantitative and the qualitative elements of care.

Triangulation

As we have seen in the book so far, the different research methodologies and associated methods all have their own advantages and disadvantages. Given each methodology and method has its weaknesses, it makes some sense for researchers to employ a variety of approaches within their research in order to minimise the impact of these failings. As early as 1959, Campbell and Fiske noted the main benefit of using triangulation of methods in research is to be certain that the findings of a study are not purely the result of the method used to collect the data. For example, one of the weaknesses associated with narrative data collection methods is that people can tell the researcher whatever they want, and the researcher has no way of knowing if what they say is, in fact, true. The weakness of an observation might be that the observer sees only what individuals are doing and how they are doing it, without understanding why they are acting in that manner. Taken together, therefore, observation and interviews (as often seen in ethnographic participant observation; see page 70) can act in a complementary manner, allowing subjects of research both to demonstrate they act in a certain way and to explain what motivates them to do so. Understanding action, and motivation for action, can be important in the management of change and the advancement of practice, as the development of practice requires nurses both to change what they do and to understand why they are changing.

The collection of data using two or more methods, or indeed methodologies, therefore gives a more rounded, or complete, picture of the activity someone is undertaking. The data collected using triangulation are sometimes described as being richer or deeper than the data collected by the use of one method alone. There are also times, however, when the data collected may appear contradictory, and significant discernment is needed on the part of the researchers to understand why this might have occurred, and how it might be overcome in the analysis and explanation of the findings. For example, when a relative claims to be concerned about the care of their loved one, but then is seen manhandling them rather than using modern safe people-handling techniques, it can be difficult to know whether they do not actually care or whether they are ignorant of the correct way to move people.

As well as collecting data in more than one way – for example, using qualitative and quantitative techniques, sometimes, confusingly, called **mixed methods research** – triangulation in research can be achieved by two or more researchers collecting data on the same phenomenon using the same, or broadly similar, methods. This technique might be useful in observational research – for example, where there may be differences, or discrepancies, in what people notice in the same or similar situations. As such, this methodological triangulation of data collection allows researchers to test the reliability and validity of the data they are collecting.

Activity 6.1 Communication

The purpose of triangulation is to improve upon perspective, to understand an issue from more than one view and therefore to gain insights that may not be readily available if only one approach to the research is used. To understand this, think about what it means to you as a nurse to provide care for an identified patient recovering from surgery or on the ward with a medical condition.

(Continued)

Triangulation of research methods also has the potential effect of reducing the amount of bias within a study. Bias can arise out of the ways in which data are collected – for example, power imbalances within a focus group can lead to the views of the most powerful becoming more dominant. Such **measurement biases** can be overcome if more than one method of collecting the data is used (for example, a questionnaire or survey being applied as well). Other forms of bias include **response bias**, when individuals answer in a manner that they believe the researcher wants them to (the Hawthorne effect). The collection of data in another manner, perhaps anonymously, may help overcome such biases.

Sampling bias is another frequent problem in studies that seek to gain insights into the understandings or beliefs of large populations. The use of a single method of data collection such as online surveys may exclude people who do not have access to the internet. Triangulating data collection methods by also undertaking face-to-face interviews in the street may serve to decrease sampling bias in a survey that uses the internet as a means of data collection.

Central to the success of the use of triangulation is the need for thought to be given to what problems, or potential problems, the use of triangulated data collection techniques can solve, and what combination of methodologies or methods will best serve to reduce the weakness of any particular approach.

For example, the weakness associated with randomised controlled trials is that they tend to collect quantitative objective data that do not recognise the individuality of the participants or their experience. Increasingly, therefore, medical research into the use of new drugs or interventions has started to include the collection of data about quality of life. While this is not perhaps the truest use of triangulation in research (as quality-of-life data tend to be collected using quantitative questionnaires), it does acknowledge that the experience of care, for example, taking a new medication or undergoing a new intervention, has to be one that has positive benefits for the patient. These benefits must accrue not only from the medical but also from the human point of view.

Berk et al. (2015) argue that the use of qualitative research methodologies to complement quantitative data collection in clinical trials of medications for psychiatric disorders helps in the generation of hypotheses for testing in subsequent randomised clinical trials, especially since, as they claim, advances in the development of medications for many mental health disorders have stalled. This proposition makes considerable sense since, as we have already discussed, qualitative research is generally inductive and quantitative deductive, with inductive being idea creating and deductive idea testing.

What is noteworthy is that for a drug or intervention to be of benefit to people, it must be not only effective but also acceptable to the people affected by it. Taub et al. (2021) illustrate this point well in their paper which discusses the need for anti-psychotic medication not only to be effective, but also safe, tolerable and acceptable in terms of side effects, etc., if adherence is to be improved.

There are a number of approaches to triangulation that all serve not only to enrich the quality of the data collected but also to verify that the data are a true reflection of reality (i.e. valid), as the participants see and experience it. These include layering data collection so that the different approaches to data collection become progressively more detailed or probing in what they seek to elicit. For example, a brief questionnaire might lead to a focus group, which might lead to a one-to-one interview. Using such techniques not only allows the richness of the data collected to be increased but also enables compensation for weaknesses of the individual methods. An example might include understanding the quality of life of patients on dialysis. A questionnaire could be used to elicit some quantitative data. These data might then be explored in the focus group setting where participants could elaborate on some of the issues raised in the questionnaire. Further individuals, perhaps those most or least typical in their contribution in the focus group, might be interviewed one to one to gain more, and different (perhaps more sensitive or personal), details.

Lorhan et al. (2015) used a review of published autobiographical data of cancer patients' experiences of care, interviews and focus groups with patients, and focus groups with volunteers and staff, to help understand both the unmet needs of patients with cancer being treated in one institution and the role that volunteers might play in meeting some of these needs. The triangulation of the methods allowed the researchers to identify patients' needs, how the volunteers met some of these needs, what gaps were left in care, how volunteers ought to be screened and ideas for more collaboration between professionals and volunteers. This study demonstrates two forms of triangulation – the use of more than one study sample group (in this case patients, volunteers and professionals) and the use of three data-collecting methods (autobiography, interview and focus groups). These two forms of triangulation help give more credence to the ideas established by the research by arriving at them in more than one way and from more than one point of view.

In their study to evaluate the reasons for seeking care among people with lower urinary tract symptoms, Griffith et al. (2018) used both an interview method and the application of a validated tool to examine the association between symptom frequency and 'bother'. They found that, in both the interview setting and using the Lower Urinary Tract Symptoms tool, the frequency with which individuals experienced symptoms was closely associated with how much bother they experienced from the symptoms. This study demonstrates that a qualitative interview and a quantitative application of a 'qualitative' tool confirm each other's findings.

As well as methodological and methods-based triangulation, there can also be theoretical triangulation within a study. Theoretical triangulation occurs when the underlying philosophy of the research is informed by more than one school of thought. For example, the **structuralist** view of ward life may be more focused on the nurses or the patients as a group in terms of the relationships between them and how they interact. From a structuralist viewpoint, the culture of an organisation is understood through studying the policies, management structures and designated roles that influence the relationships of people within it. Whereas, from an **interactionist** viewpoint, the culture of an organisation is understood through studying how people interact in relationships, negotiate their respective roles and comply with or deviate from what is expected of them.

Theoretical triangulation is therefore about exploring a concept, experience, attitude or interaction from more than one standpoint and, like methodological triangulation, it is about gaining multiple insights into the same issue by taking more than one philosophical starting point. Practically, this is achieved by using more than one research methodology and associated methods. Ones that allow structuralist exploration might include applying an ethnographic methodology or the collection of data by observation or focus groups, while interactionist examination might require individual interviews.

Fundamental to the success of triangulation is that the blend of approaches used to collect data complement and supplement each other in a reasoned and thought-out way. This requires the researcher to have a good grasp of the pros and cons of each of the methodologies and methods that can be used in nursing research, and to be open to the idea that no single approach to research in nursing practice can be said to hold all of the answers.

Concept summary: triangulation

It may be helpful to use the metaphor of a map to think about triangulation of research methodologies and methods. If you want to tell other people where you are, providing only the longitudinal co-ordinates is of little help. But when you provide the latitudinal co-ordinates as well, it is easy for others to find you. In a similar sense, the use of triangulated research methods enhances the ability of researchers not only to find out in more detail the reality of whatever they are researching but to communicate to others these findings with increased accuracy and confidence.

So, we can view the use of triangulated research as a means of adding a further dimension to research. This additional dimension improves validity by demonstrating that what has been measured is actually a good representation of what we set out to measure. Triangulation also improves reliability by demonstrating that what has been measured and characterised in the research has been shown to hold true when measured in more than one way.

Evaluation research

Evaluation research as a methodology is used to measure the worth or merit of something. It employs any of the methods highlighted in the previous chapters. The key difference lies in the fact that evaluation research occurs within an organisational context, such as a hospital, ward or healthcare team, and it therefore requires the researcher to exercise great diplomatic skills. The nature of evaluative research is such that it requires the involvement of multiple stakeholders whose social, political, professional and personal sensitivities have not only to be recognised but also to be respected.

Evaluation research is a systematic undertaking, and the object of the evaluation can be defined in many different ways. As such, the object of the evaluation may be a programme of care, a care process, the functioning of the ward or care area, the people within the organisation or team, the key activities of the team or organisation or any combination of the above.

Much of the literature in this area reflects that the evaluation aspect of evaluation research often has as much – if not more – to do with the quality and usefulness of the data it collects as with the usefulness or merit of the objects, people or processes it is evaluating.

The goal of evaluation research is, therefore, to derive findings that can be used to drive change. The change that ensues has to be driven by the findings of the evaluation and seen to be driven by in-depth empirical investigation of the object of evaluation and not the 'second-hand' application of evidence derived from some study, regardless of the presumed generalisability of the study.

Activity 6.2   Critical thinking

Consider some of the questions we have asked about the adoption of research in the area in which you work. What are the issues that derive from research that is undertaken in a different social, political or cultural setting? How do these affect the applicability of research to different settings? How might focused evaluation research be helpful in overcoming these issues?

There are some possible answers at the end of the chapter.

You might rightly question why evaluation of a service or process should fall under the umbrella of research rather than audit. Booth (2009) provides four good reasons why evaluation through research rather than evaluative audit is important.

1. Service evaluation tends to be more descriptive and less analytical when undertaken as an audit.

2. Evaluation research helps in the pursuit of an actual answer to the question of quality rather than the generation of further questions that might need further research and do not resolve issues in practice.

3. Evaluation research is more likely to generate statistically tested outcomes that show cause and effect than a local evaluation audit, which will produce statistics that describe only the magnitude of the issue.

4. Evaluation research is more likely to generate findings that can be applied elsewhere (they are generalisable) than a purely locally based evaluation of a service, thus adding to the body of knowledge in an area for the benefit of all.

The use of evaluation research, therefore, has many benefits over and above a pure service evaluation/audit. Service evaluations by their very nature can be threatening to the people who provide the service. They have the potential to discover that the service provided needs improvement or that it is failing in some areas. Undertaking evaluation research, on the other hand, not only provides credibility for the methods used to collect the data, through the application of rigorous research methods, but also means that the ethical principles that apply to the generation of knowledge through research are adhered to (Kara, 2018).

The necessity for evaluation research is well established in the healthcare setting where the worth of what we do as nurses needs to be demonstrated. Not only is this a matter of the clinical, ethical and human imperative of doing the best for our patients, but it also arises out of the need to demonstrate that we are making the best use of the resources available – understood holistically, therefore, evaluation research allows health and social care professionals to demonstrate the evidence base for their practice. Given the diversity of reasons for undertaking evaluation research, it follows that the methods employed within evaluation research are not restricted to either qualitative or quantitative approaches; rather, the methods that best fit the needs and purposes of the evaluation are applied. As such, evaluation research, with its focus on assessing the usefulness or value of something, can draw on methods from either, or both, research paradigms.

In their evaluation study of the perceived ease of use of a prototype reusable pen injector delivering recombinant human growth hormone, Sauer and Abbotts (2018) demonstrated acceptance of the device and its ease of use among patients, caregivers and healthcare professionals. The study assessed ease of use and acceptability via semi-structured interviews but only included patients who had experience of using the device for more than six months and professionals who had trained people to use it and saw more than four users of growth hormone a month. This study shows how evaluation research is used to examine a change in clinical practice, and that the participants need to be purposively sampled. It also demonstrated some triangulation in that the acceptability of the device was demonstrated in both the patient and professional participants and it was undertaken in five countries.

Starting evaluation research

Evaluating the context within which an evaluation takes place is perhaps the most important step in the evaluation research process and is a step that is often undertaken implicitly but not discussed within either the research or the research textbooks.

Context evaluation requires the environment within which the evaluation is to take place to be fully explored and understood before the process of evaluation takes place. There are many factors that impact on the evaluation of the delivery of care. These include issues from the social, political and economic climate within which care is provided, as well as the characteristics of the people involved in the delivery and receipt of care (as we saw in our example above).

As such, an evaluation of the context of care will identify the limitations that are placed on the process of the evaluation research. Evaluating the context of the evaluation research also enables the researcher to identify the people who are the stakeholders – people affecting and affected (e.g. caregivers and people in the receipt of care) by whatever is being evaluated. Understanding the context of the research, and the nature and variety of the stakeholders, will enable researchers to make informed choices about the approaches they will adopt in the evaluation research study.

Types of evaluation research

Needs assessment

Needs assessment might be used to evaluate whether there is a need for the provision of a new programme of care or a change to a programme currently being provided. The needs assessment may then be used both to substantiate the need for the creation of a new or changed programme and also in the design of a programme. Needs assessments are not an evaluation of an existing service or programme of care, they are a means of identifying and quantifying the potential need for a future service.

A needs assessment may be useful in helping to gain approval and funding for a new service. Its purpose is to help identify what needs the new service can be used to meet, as well as identifying those people who might most benefit from the new service.

For example, it is well documented that the uptake of haemodialysis services is highest in areas where a dialysis unit is situated. This tends to suggest that if people live some distance from a dialysis unit, they opt not to have haemodialysis, are not given the option of haemodialysis or choose peritoneal dialysis (usually home-based). A needs assessment of the requirement for a new dialysis unit might therefore take into account the positioning of existing units as well as the numbers and geographical locations of people with known end-stage kidney disease. It would also consider the demographic characteristics of the population within a location, especially where these characteristics are known to increase the risks for developing renal disease.

Process evaluation

Process evaluations are designed to demonstrate whether a new or changed programme has been implemented in the manner in which it was conceived, as well as examining whether the people accessing the service believe it to be of benefit. The sort of data collected in a process evaluation may include the number of people who use the service and what services they actually received. There is also a qualitative element to this evaluation in that the users of the new service are asked to evaluate its usefulness to them.

For example, in the case of the new dialysis unit described above, there would be evaluations of the numbers of people using the service and what service they actually receive, as well as the impact of the delivery of the new service on patients' perception of the quality of the care provided to them. Such an evaluation would take into account both quantitative and qualitative data, which could be collected using a variety of methods.

In their process evaluation of the predictive value of using multiple mini-interviews as part of a values-based recruitment exercise for pre-registration healthcare professionals, Callwood et al. (2018) used statistical models to demonstrate the value of a seven-station mini-interview process for predicting practice outcomes at the end of the first year. This study demonstrated that changes to the recruitment process for healthcare professional students using multiple mini-interviews might be useful in aiding recruitment processes to be values-driven.

Formative evaluation

Much in the same way that the progress of student nurses is evaluated part-way through their time on a placement in order to inform them what they need to do to improve, formative evaluations of a new service use data gathered during the early phases of the service to help inform and modify the way in which the service develops. Plainly, these data will include both quantitative and qualitative elements and will reflect the nature of the service being provided.

For example, soon after opening a new dialysis unit, an evaluation of the uptake of the service against that predicted in the initial needs assessment would give some idea of whether the new service is likely to meet its aspirations.

Summative evaluation

Sometimes referred to as an outcome evaluation, summative evaluation is used to measure whether the aims of the service provided have actually been met. This is, again, similar to the summative evaluation given to student nurses at the end of their clinical placement, where they reflect on the objectives that they had been set to see if they have managed to achieve them during the placement.

What is clear is that summative evaluation research looks back at the objectives and aims set at the start of the programme or service and uses these as a benchmark against which delivery is measured. For example, an evaluation of a new dialysis service some months after it opened would give an indication of whether it has progressed from the formative evaluation towards meeting the targets set for the service.

Efficiency evaluation

These evaluations are sometimes called 'cost-effectiveness' or 'cost–benefit valuations'. The purpose of efficiency evaluation research is to examine whether the new service provides good value for money in meeting the objectives that were set for it at the start. For example, a new dialysis unit might be evaluated to see whether it is saving transport costs by treating patients nearer to home, and whether these savings offset the costs of providing the service in the additional location. The important issues with this type of evaluation are not always purely financial but, rather, whether the benefits of the service match up to, or preferably surpass, the money spent. In the case of the haemodialysis patient who has to dialyse three times a week for three to four hours, this benefit may accrue from considerably reduced travelling times and a more personal service in a smaller unit.

Utilisation evaluation

The final type of evaluation research discussed here is utilisation evaluation research. The purpose of this type of evaluation research is to appraise whether the evaluations of the new service or programme have actually been used. It is clear that this type of evaluation research seeks to ascertain whether good practice in the delivery of care persists beyond the end of a programme of initial evaluation.

In nursing we are all aware of the fact that standards and practices change over time and often not always for the right reasons. Many useful evaluations of services are dropped because policy makers or managers have decided that they cannot be afforded or because the levels of motivation within the service delivery team are low.

Utilisation evaluations seek to reinvigorate services by reconnecting the people delivering the service with the quality measures of that service. The purpose is to ensure that the findings of previous evaluation, audit and research are being used to inform the delivery of care.

Utilisation evaluation research is potentially an important aspect of clinical effectiveness and governance. The focus of utilisation evaluation research on measuring the uptake and utilisation of previous findings makes it a clear source of information to inform evidence-based nursing practice in a way that reflects the proficiencies highlighted at the start of the chapter. As such, it is potentially an important research tool for the clinically based nurse.

Action research

Key features

Action research delivers exactly what it says. Action research is research *in and on* action. The purpose of the enquiry of action research is improvement in the quality of the actions and performance of an organisation, team or individual. The central tenet of the action research approach is that it involves, or preferably is driven by, the people whom it most affects – the key stakeholders – who in the context of this book are often the nurses who work in a specific team or organisation and their patients.

Because of the team approach to undertaking action research, it is often termed a collaborative enquiry. The scope of the team involved in the collaborative enquiry extends beyond the immediate team to all of the individuals who affect, and are affected by, what the team does.

Activity 6.3   Reflection

Thinking about the scope of the enquiry associated with action research, take a few moments to think about all of the people who are involved in the delivery and receipt of care where you work at present. Be careful to include all of the people whose roles, however menial they may appear, have an impact not only on the quality of what you do in terms of patients' physical outcomes but also on their experience of care.

There are some possible answers at the end of the chapter.

The purpose and focus of action research is to produce realistic and sustainable improvements in the delivery of care in the setting in which the action research takes place. It allows the providers of the care to reflect on what they do, how they do it and why. It also allows them to explore potential new methods for the delivery of care along with the potential benefits and pitfalls that might accrue from this. The collaborative nature of the process means that the insights and ideas generated are open for sharing and discussion with all of the stakeholders in the process, and the decisions that are therefore made about changes to, and improvements in, practice are, potentially, reached through true consensus.

In their action research project, Kemp et al. (2018) sought to develop a national standard for midwifery mentorship in Uganda. The project was built around three action cycles: participatory workshops, individual twinning arrangements between UK and Ugandan midwives and peer exchange visits. The findings from these interactions were used to inform a capacity-building programme specifically to design the standard for midwifery mentorship. This study demonstrated action research features in that it was built around the creation of a programme to develop a standard; it involved multiple strands of interaction and enquiry; and it involved the stakeholders in the process.

The British tradition of action research echoes the view of action research as research that is focused on the direct improvement of practice. This tradition is firmly grounded in reflection. Classic action research is described by Carr and Kemmis (1986, p162) as *simply a form of self-reflective enquiry undertaken by participants in social situations in order to improve the rationality and justice of their own practices, their understanding of these practices, and the situations in which the practices are carried out.*

As such, this form of action research is attractive to nurses, who are practised in reflection from working in the academic and clinical setting.

The action research cycle

The need for an action research project often arises out of the realisation that there is an issue in practice that needs addressing but for which there appears to be no readily identifiable solution.

Lewin (1946), who coined the phrase 'action research', created the cycle of action research (Figure 6.1), which is still guiding many action researchers to date. Many researchers refer to the cycle as the methodology which guides action research. The adoption of the cycle as a map for action research is, however, probably a misinterpretation of the purpose of the cycle, which is more of a guide than a methodological blueprint.

The recurring cycles of action research produce spirals of action, with the researcher re-entering the cycle as many times as required to address new issues that arise during the implementation of the action phases.

This action research cycle is often stated as being 'reflect, plan, act, observe, reflect' and, as such, mirrors in many ways the nursing process of 'assess, plan, implement and evaluate'. The starting point for a piece of action research can be any point within this cycle. For instance, the realisation of the need for change might arise out of reflection on a clinical incident or issue, or the need to implement a new externally imposed process, policy or procedure that requires some changes in the way in which the team or organisation works.

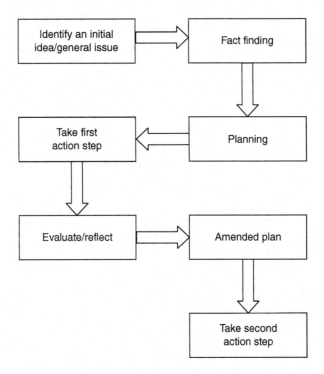

Figure 6.1   The action research cycle

Source: adapted from Lewin (1946).

In their action research study, Paltved et al. (2015) set out to transform interprofessional practice on a surgical ward. More specifically, they explored professional identity and clinical decision making, developed a model for changing the way professionals worked together and evaluated the change model and the process of action research. The study involved 60 doctors and nurses and the use of a number of research data-collecting methods. Together, the participants **co-created** their own vision of interprofessional working and used this to drive changes to improve patient care. In this study we see action research demonstrated in the way the participants identify the issues of identity and decision making, develop new ways of working and then evaluate these new ways of working. Presumably the participants will continue in the cycle to improve patient care in their facility in an ongoing fashion.

What makes action research such a challenge to undertake is that there is often more than one spiral of action underway at any time. This means that researchers engaged in action research may be reflecting on the impact of one action while simultaneously implementing another.

The process of action research relies more on democracy, reflexivity, change and collaboration than slavishly following a prescribed methodology. Because of its agenda of effecting meaningful and lasting change, there is a requirement that action research meets the needs of all of the people involved and that all the people it affects are involved (democracy and collaboration).

Given the involvement of the researchers in the process and because the very presence of the researchers has an impact on the process, there is a requirement that, as well as being reflective, the researchers are also reflexive. Reflexivity requires researchers to be open to and understand the impact of their presence, their actions and the choices that they make on the process of the research.

Data collection methods

The methods used for the collection of data within action research are restricted only by the imagination and skills of the people undertaking the research. As a methodology, action research is not bounded by the philosophies and conventions associated with the quantitative or qualitative paradigms, although some studies identify themselves as being influenced by a particular paradigm or ideology such as feminism.

Data collection within action research requires not only that the issue under investigation is understood but also that data are collected so that the nature of the plan, actions derived from the plan and the subsequent evaluation and reflection on the action are coherently and comprehensively understood.

This means that data collection within action research is driven more by the nature of the individual questions that arise than by the paradigm within which it sits. Typical data collection strategies, therefore, include surveys, questionnaires, interviews, focus groups, examination of existing records and observation. As within the traditional paradigms and their associated methodologies and methods, thought needs to be given to which approaches to data collection are likely to produce the data that are needed to meet the aims of the research. An action research project is not restricted to the use of one method of data collection; rather, the different phases of the action research process may require different methodological approaches and methods of data collection, depending on the particular problem being addressed.

Rapid appraisal

Rapid appraisal is an increasingly popular qualitative methodology which investigates phenomena at community level (Bowling, 2014) using methods which emerge as the question being asked is answered. Rapid appraisal is used to gain insight into the collective view of a community (e.g. in a location, a profession or other group) about its needs.

Sometimes rapid appraisal is embedded within action research as the means of identifying areas for change. Rapid appraisal is similar to ethnography but takes place, as the name suggests, over a very short period of time. As a methodology, rapid appraisal is often used to evaluate a project formatively (that is before it is fully embedded) to ensure it is on track, to aid decision making in the absence of more substantial methodologies (especially when time is tight), and to inform the design of subsequent research (USAID, 2010).

Rapid appraisal methods were widely used as a means of evaluating service provision and staff experiences of working with COVID-positive patients during the COVID-19 pandemic (Vindrola-Padros et al., 2020)

Rapid appraisal seeks to investigate whatever it finds. As data emerge from the enquiry it is then tested by asking the same question in a different way, or perhaps by using a different method, making rapid appraisal truly an inductive and iterative research method in which data findings are triangulated. Data for rapid appraisals are collected via a variety of means, including workshops, postal surveys, semi-structured interviews, reviews of existing records and area or team profiling (Ellis, 2018).

The fact that rapid appraisal uses multiple methods adds to the faith which can be placed in the validity of its findings. Rapid appraisal is also not a solitary undertaking. The fact that groups of people as well as more than one researcher are involved in data collection adds to the reliability of the methodology.

Activity 6.4   Research and finding out

Go online and using a reputable bibliographic database find a research project which has used rapid appraisal as its key methodology. Within the article identify the purpose of the appraisal, the population it applies to and the methods used to collect the data. Pay special attention to the ways in which the data are analysed and used to inform subsequent phases of the appraisal.

As this is based on your own research, there is no specimen answer at the end of the chapter.

Chapter summary

This chapter has established that strict adherence to qualitative or quantitative research methodologies or single data collection methods may not always be the best approach to answering complex questions arising out of the delivery of nursing care. We have established that understanding and delivering good-quality care require us to understand not only the physical and psychological aspects of care but also the emotional aspects and how the care is experienced.

Triangulation has been highlighted as one way in which the philosophy, methodology and methods of research can be reconciled so that more than one dimension of a problem can be explored. We see that, by viewing a research issue from more than one standpoint, the understanding that can be gained is both deeper and better defined. We have also seen how

(Continued)

(Continued)

triangulation can be used to increase the faith which can be placed in the outcomes from a study, or not, and how it can add precision to findings from research.

We have seen that evaluation research allows for the appraisal of a team, an organisation or a programme of care. We have seen that evaluation is bounded to a time and a place and is designed to answer questions about the area being researched. Evaluation research is therefore portrayed as a helpful means of collecting data that are perhaps more meaningful than those collected by some forms of clinical audit, in effecting meaningful change.

We also discussed the nature of action research and rapid appraisals – unusual among the research methodologies in that the subjects of the research are also intimately involved in the research. We have seen that action research and rapid appraisals rarely follow a predetermined methodology; rather, they are responsive to their own findings and adapt as they progress.

Activities: brief outline answers

Activity 6.2   Critical thinking (page 145)

Research undertaken in different settings is affected by the demographic make-up of the population from which the sample for the research is drawn. The way in which the sample is selected also has potential to affect the applicability of the research findings to the clinical setting. Evaluation research undertaken in the area in which the findings are to be applied overcomes these issues as it draws its sample from the same population the research will take place in.

Activity 6.3   Reflection (page 150)

Potential stakeholders in action research in the care setting are:

- nurses;
- students;
- doctors;
- allied health professionals;
- support staff;
- patients;
- patients' relatives;
- voluntary staff;
- the community at large.

Further reading

Creswell, JW and Plano Clark, VL (2018) *Designing and Conducting Mixed Methods Research* (3rd edn). London: Sage.

Lathlean, J (2015) Evaluation research, in Gerrish, K and Lathlean, J (eds) *The Research Process in Nursing* (7th edn). Oxford: Wiley-Blackwell.

McNiff, J (2014) *Writing and Doing Action Research*. London: Sage.

A comprehensive and user-friendly guide to action research.

Meyer, J and Cooper, J (2015) Action research, in Gerrish, K and Lathlean, J (eds) *The Research Process in Nursing* (7th edn). Oxford: Wiley-Blackwell.

Pope, C and Mays, N (2020) *Foundations of Nursing Research* (4th edn). London: Wiley-Blackwell.

See Chapter 12 on mixed methods and Chapter 14 on participatory research.

Streubert, HJ and Carpenter, DR (2010) *Qualitative Research in Nursing: Advancing the Humanistic Imperative* (5th edn). London: Wolters Kluwer Health/Lippincott Williams & Wilkins.

Chapter 15, 'Triangulation as a qualitative research strategy', gives a brief but informative overview of this subject area.

Useful websites

www.carn.org.uk/ The Collaborative Action Research Network (see the 'resources' tab for other useful links).

www.jeanmcniff.com Look under the 'booklet' tab for a brief and simple-to-read introduction to action research from a leading exponent of it.

www.rapidresearchandevaluation.com Look at the resources and publications here to find out more about rapid appraisal research.

Chapter 7 · Using research

Introduction

So far this book has introduced you to the main paradigms, methodologies, methods and terminology associated with undertaking research in a nursing and healthcare context. For some readers this will have been a journey of necessity, for example because you are taking a research module at university, while for others this will have been purely through an interest in the subject area of research; in reality the reason for writing this book has been to address, at least in part, both of these. Of course, the main motive for being interested in research and research practice for all exponents of health and social care, and the reason this book was written, is the recognition of the positive impact that research can have on the health and well-being of the people we care for.

In this deliberately brief chapter, we will consider how we might use the content of the rest of the book to address a number of your needs as a student both in the immediate term (to pass assignments and plan projects) and in the long term to deliver informed and judicious care.

Why research is important

Elsewhere in this series Ellis (2019) presents an extended argument as to why the use of evidence in nursing practice is important. There are some key reasons why the use of evidence-based practice is important that are worth reiterating here.

The key starting point is to understand knowledge changes over time. What we think we 'know' today might be shown to be wrong tomorrow as human understanding and technologies for understanding the world develop. This means we cannot rest on our laurels: we have to engage with nursing as a lifelong learning exercise, developing what we do and how we do it to reflect the needs of society, patients and clients as well as the current state of knowledge. In some cases this will be by appreciating and adopting a new approach to treating some disease or disability (as we saw in the quantitative chapters), while in others (as we have seen in the chapters on qualitative research) it will be about understanding how people experience their treatment and the care we provide. Either way, as individuals we can make the choice either just to adopt the changes because we have been told to do so, or we can try to understand, or indeed introduce, the changes ourselves.

Activity 7.1   Reflection

Review the box 'Concept summary: empiricism' in Chapter 1 (page 5) and consider how changes in knowledge over time might create an argument for continuing to engage with lifelong learning and evidence-based practice.

As the answer is based on your own reflection, there is no outline answer at the end of the chapter.

However we choose to view it, using research is an integral part of the role of the nurse. There is a moral imperative for us to provide the best care we can for our clients and patients, and this means at a minimum being able to understand what is good and what is bad in the research we read, and therefore how much faith we place in it prior to adopting it in practice. This has been the purpose of this book: not to teach you how to critique research, but to provide you with the understanding of research so that you can apply this understanding to critiquing. This moral imperative reflects the need for nurses to also make the best use of the resources available to them.

A good deal of what health and social care practitioners do is not research-based, but then most health and social care commentators now agree that evidence-based practice, widely agreed to be the proper way to provide care, is not, cannot and will never be entirely research-driven (Ellis, 2019). There are a number of good reasons why research and evidence-based care are not synonymous:

- Not everything can be researched.
- Not everything has been researched.
- Not all situations are identical and therefore existing research may not apply.
- Research outcomes only apply to broadly similar situations.
- People have the right to make non-research-based choices.

Activity 7.2   Critical thinking

Consider the above list of reasons as to why some care cannot be informed by research and identify the ideas and concepts which you have read in this book which underpin these.

There is an outline answer at the end of the chapter.

What the above list demonstrates is that there are many influences on the decisions we make as nurses and there are many reasons why research may not always inform practice. Ellis (2019) lists a number of influences on the decisions we make in practice:

- research evidence;
- practice knowledge;
- experience;
- policy;
- resources;
- patient preference;
- views of other professionals;
- ethics;
- law.

Evidently, these influences are of differing levels of importance depending on the scenario to which they are being applied but, and this is an important but, of the influences on practice, research evidence is, when of good quality, the most credible and readily justifiable. Each of the other influences on practice, while important as a consideration for how and why we might act, is open to opinion and individual interpretation.

The NMC Standards of Proficiency for Registered Nurses highlighted at the start of this chapter exhort us to act 'as a role model for others in providing evidence based person-centred care'.

These are lofty ideals and, as we move further into the era of increased professionalisation of nursing, with the attendant need to role model, and to supervise the work of other practitioners, the importance of these standards of proficiency becomes more evident.

The rest of this chapter will explore a little of how research can be used to inform both practice situations and academic work. The reader is advised to look elsewhere for more in-depth discussion and analysis of the other available, and valid, approaches to decision making (see further reading at the end of this chapter).

Using research to inform practice

Getting research into practice involves a number of key steps. One of the first things we need to be clear about is the fact that not all research is good, not all research comes to the right conclusions and not all research will necessarily apply to the situation before us.

Moule (2021) suggests a very useful route plan for the adoption of evidence in practice using five distinct but connected stages. Of note, each of the stages requires the nurse to be critical not only of the evidence presented but also within each of the stages of the process.

1. Identify a problem from practice and turn it into a specific question.

2. Find the best available evidence that relates to the question, usually by systematically searching the literature.

3. Appraise the evidence.

4. Identify the best evidence alongside the patient's needs and preferences.

5. Evaluate the effect of applying the evidence.

The rest of this chapter will essentially use this five-stage model to inform our thinking about how we might use research either for an academic undertaking or to improve practice.

Stages 1–3 provide a useful blueprint for many academic undertakings such as critiquing literature within an evidence-based practice or research module or in the process of designing a piece of research. Good academic practice in general requires the explicit and thoughtful use of research to inform any essay or assignment, and this will include being critical about its quality. The discussion that follows about these first three stages will therefore be helpful in the planning and execution of such undertakings, but readers are advised to look elsewhere to extend and supplement their understanding as well (see the 'Further reading' section at the end of this chapter).

Of course, not all academic work is specifically about designing or critiquing research studies; there are many other occasions when the use of research in an essay is needed. Any academic paper that has a clinical element to it should be informed by the use of research and more specifically journal-based literature. There are two good reasons for this: the first is that clinical textbooks become out of date quickly as new advances in care delivery are discovered and therefore your development as a practitioner *must* be supplemented by an understanding of current best practice. The second reason is that it demonstrates your ability to identify and engage with lifelong learning and as such will impress the marker!

As with all academic undertakings, it is not enough merely to cite or quote research; the best students will also include some description of the context of the research and perhaps a critique of the methodology/methods as well. Such critique demonstrates the ability to understand the context of research and independent thinking.

If you are considering how you might use research to inform and practise better, all five stages of the model are of benefit, and again you are advised to use further literature to inform your thinking in this area (see the 'Further reading' section at the end of this chapter).

Generating a specific question

Generating a specific question relating to a clinical situation is not always as easy as it might seem. In Chapter 1 we explored the use of the acronyms SPICE and PICO to enable us to generate questions that are clear, focused and relevant.

Once we have identified our practice problem and turned it into a useful question there is increased clarity about what exactly we are trying to achieve. For example, are we looking for a hard-and-fast scientific answer to a medical, technical or measurable issue, or are we trying to understand the opinions, attitudes or beliefs that inform a behaviour or response to treatment? This in turn helps us to identify which of the two paradigms (or potentially mixed methodology) of research we should be exploring. Table 2.3 in Chapter 2 and Table 4.1 in Chapter 4 provide some insight into the types of question different research approaches might be able to answer.

Finding the best available evidence

When we have a useful question we are ready to take the next step in the process, which is to search the literature (see the chapter 'Sources of knowledge for evidence-based care' in Ellis, 2019).

There are some important issues about how and where we might find evidence that is worth considering here. Students and nurses should always consider that, just because something is in print, on the web or has been told to you, it does not mean it is necessarily right. The first clue we might gather as to the usefulness of a source of information is the quality of the resource itself. Looking for information to inform practice in a general newspaper or an unmoderated website is most certainly not a good idea. Quality sources of information for nursing include those websites and journals that are **peer-reviewed** (that is, where the content has been reviewed by other specialists in the field to confirm its quality). For the most part, such sources will be aimed at a professional audience, which may include nurses and other health and social care professionals; this is, of course, subject-dependent.

Activity 7.4 Evidence-based practice and research

Take the time to find a newspaper and identify a health-related story in it. Read the story in detail, taking note of the use of health language and ideas and the interpretations placed

(Continued)

(Continued)

on these. Now go online to a professional site or look in a professional journal or book for information on the same topic, taking note of how the information is presented and the conclusions the authors come to. Compare and contrast the two ways of covering the issue. Consider what might happen to healthcare provision if policy and practice were based on newspaper-style interpretations of health issues and stories.

There is an outline answer at the end of the chapter.

Good-quality journals can be searched using bibliographic databases such as CINAHL (Cumulative Index of Nursing and Allied Health Literature) and the British Nursing Index. Using the terminology identified in the generation of the question is step 1, followed by the use of other key words that are focused on the topic in hand. Learning to search bibliographic databases effectively is a good skill to have for either academic or clinical purposes; all universities and many hospital libraries will provide workshops on how to do this effectively.

Appraising the evidence

This is the real crux of the whole process. Understanding research requires engagement with reading and comprehension of the research process. Whatever you are reading research for, the stages involved in its appraisal, and the tools you will need, remain the same. As well as using a critiquing framework (see, for example, Ellis (2019), a snippet of which is provided later) for effective evaluation of research, you will also need to hand at least one good research textbook, which you can use as a reference as to what good research looks like.

The access to good quality critiquing tools online is improving all the time. The Critical Appraisal Skills Programme (CASP) is one such website providing free access to critiquing tools (see useful websites at the end of this chapter). On the CASP website you will find a variety of checklists which can be used for critically appraising different types of research; similarly, the Joanna Briggs Institute (JBI) (see useful websites at the end of this chapter) also hosts a suite of critical appraisal tools.

One of the key errors students make when critiquing research is to think the use of a word in research is synonymous with the use of the word in everyday life. This means they often fail to appreciate what a framework is asking them to do – *critique*. For example, the use of the term 'bias' in research is, as we have seen elsewhere in the book, very specific, therefore applying the term in its everyday sense is not what is required. So tip two for effective critiquing is to use a glossary (like the one in this book) to ensure you understand and apply critiquing terms correctly. Getting the critique right will also impact on the potential clinical application of a research paper where, for example, selection biases may mean that a study is not pertinent to the patients you are caring for – that is, the findings are not generalisable or transferable.

Activity 7.5   Evidence-based practice and research

Consider the use of the terms validity, reliability and bias in everyday life. What do they mean and in what contexts might you use them? Now research the meaning of validity, reliability and bias in relation to research – what do they mean and in what contexts do they apply? You might like to use the Glossary in this book, as well as the Index to return to where these terms are discussed, to help you with this exercise.

As this activity is based on your own research, there is no outline answer at the end of the chapter.

This idea of the use of research terminology in critiquing leads us to a third tip in relation to successful critiquing, especially in the academic sense. In an essay or other written assignment you only have one opportunity to get your point across and to let the marker know that you know what you are talking about, so to ensure you make this communication effectively it is useful to *define* your terms, *reference* the definition and then *apply* the definition to the critique.

Concept summary: defining, referencing and applying a research definition

In an essay or other written assignment, you might say that in qualitative research the term 'trustworthiness' is used to refer to the quality of the procedures used in the process of undertaking the research; this is your *definition*. You might then *reference* this definition to a good-quality, pertinent research textbook. You would then *apply* the definition to the critique by saying whatever it is you wanted to say about the quality of the research procedures used in the research in question.

In the academic sense it is then important to critique the elements of the paper you are asked to critique; no more and no less. Often academic critiques focus on elements of the question asked, the paradigm, methodology and methods chosen. A good critique will examine each of these in turn with reference to a research textbook (or preferably more than one) to define what they are and the pros and cons of each. The very best students will also define terms like paradigm, methodology and method as part of the critique in order to demonstrate to the marker that they know exactly what they are doing and that they understand the research process in some detail.

Again in the academic setting, it may be important to suggest alternative ways of answering the same question (although for practical applications of research critiquing this may not be so important). So, for example, the critiquing framework by Ellis (2019) suggests asking the following questions.

- Given the methodology identified (if any), do the research data collection methods fit?
- Even if yes, are there alternative methods that might be appropriate as well?

Providing a full answer to these questions demonstrates to the marker that you understand not only how to critique what is in front of you, but also the range of techniques available to collect data in similar situations, that is to say, you understand the broader research process. A good example of this would be using focus groups to collect data about people's experiences of care, which might prove as useful as collecting the same data via interviews.

Using the best evidence and considering patient preference

In the practice setting the use of evidence is about the way in which we, as nurses, respond to the reality of the patient's situation. That means our critique of evidence provides only one step of the process in clinical decision making.

Perhaps the most widely quoted definition comes from Sackett et al. (1996, p71), who defined evidence-based medicine as:

> the conscientious, explicit and judicious use of current best evidence in making decisions about the care of the individual patient. It means integrating individual clinical expertise with the best available external clinical evidence from systematic research.

What Sackett et al. are saying here is that we need to ensure the decisions we make are guided by thoughtful processes that are shaped by both explicit forms of evidence (such as research) and the requirements of the individual patient. It does not matter that this definition is about medicine, since the same ideas translate to the adoption of evidence in nursing or any other form of professional practice.

Of course, we have to make other judgements about research and other forms of evidence in the context of our practice before we consider if, when and how we might apply it. Øvretveit (2017) asks the pertinent question, *Would it work here?* In asking this question, Øvretveit is reminding us that, while research is a useful indicator of what good healthcare might look like, we should consider some practicalities. Some questions you might ask when considering the application of research are suggested below.

Questions to ask before adopting research-driven change

- Can we afford the change?
- What are the potential benefits to:
  - patients
  - staff
  - the organisation?

- What are the potential disadvantages to:
  - patients
  - staff
  - the organisation?

- Are the people in the research broadly similar to the people we will be applying it to?
- What might our patients (current and future) think about this?
- What are the alternatives?
- Do we have the skills necessary, or can we acquire them?
- How will we instigate the change?
- Who will lead the change?

While, in the broadest sense, these are reasonable questions to ask, we might also consider what alternatives might be in place for patients who do not want the change we are considering adopting (e.g. an alteration to a wound-dressing regime or changing the mode of delivery of a medication).

The key message here is that, while research is perhaps the most useful tool we have to inform practice, it is not an end in itself. Essentially, this means that people do not do research in healthcare for the sake of doing research, they do it to find an answer to a question which might in turn inform practice.

Research in nursing is applied in a context of human interaction and as such needs to consider ability, preference and affordability. Any adoption of research evidence into practice that does not account for these will be more likely to fail than one that does, not least because people, nurses included, are very often scared by change (for a broader discussion of this, see *Evidence-Based Practice in Nursing* (Ellis, 2019), also in this series).

Activity 7.6   Reflection

Consider a time when you had to make a change in your life. Perhaps it was moving away from home to go to university or starting on a new practice placement for the first time.

(Continued)

(Continued)

Even though these are positive events, what negative emotions did you experience? Consider also how you felt making the transition from school to university essay writing. You may have developed a style of writing for school that was effective and brought you success and now you are being asked to relearn something you thought you had already mastered; what impact did this have on how you felt about yourself and your academic ability?

As the answer is based on your own reflection, there is no outline answer at the end of the chapter.

What you might note on undertaking this reflection is that all change is associated with an emotional response. Changes that impact on how you feel about yourself and your ability can feel very alarming. The essential message here is that the adoption of evidence for practice is not purely an academic process; the need to bring people (patients and staff alike) along on the journey is as important as, if not more than, understanding the evidence itself. This bringing along, includes developing the ability to address people's fears of the unknown as well as ensuring they understand what you are trying to achieve and why this is better than what is already in place.

Patients are people, and in modern society people possess the right to make choices, even if these are considered to be *bad* ones, so part of the armoury of the evidence-based nurse is the ability to inform patients of their options and then to work *with* them to make choices that suit their individual circumstances and preferences – in this respect, research is an essential tool in the delivery of patient-centred care.

Evaluating the application of evidence

We noted early on in the chapter that providing good-quality, evidence-driven care is a moral imperative for nurses. Meeting the demands of this moral imperative requires that in the practice setting we evaluate what we have done and its effectiveness; at no time is this more important than after we have made a change to practice.

The purpose of evaluating a change is to answer the question, *Has it worked here?* In some respects evaluating the outcomes of the adoption of evidence in this way injects an air of reality into the process because it answers many of the *questions to ask* before adopting research-driven change we posed previously. Evaluation post-implementation is in many senses more realistic than asking questions before the implementation because we are measuring what *actually* happened, rather than what *might* happen.

Evaluating the implementation of research is also important because, as we have seen, research scenarios are often manipulated to suit the needs of the research itself and therefore they may not represent real life.

The process of evaluating a change is much like the process of undertaking research using the methodology of a quasi- (or natural) experiment (discussed in Chapter 4).

Considering the requirements of a natural experiment it is clear that we need to collect data both before and after a change has been implemented in order to compare and contrast two approaches to care. So, for example, if we were to alter a self-care regime we might want to measure the impact of the change on clinical staff stress as well as, perhaps, the staff-perceived experience of care giving.

Case study

Orellana-Rios et al. (2017) undertook a study to assess the effectiveness of a ten-week group programme to introduce people working in palliative care to mindfulness and compassion-oriented meditation training with a view to reducing the distress experienced in the workplace. They used validated tools to measure stress, burnout, depression, anxiety and coping methods, undertook qualitative interviews, as well as measuring serum cortisol (a good indicator of stress) both before and after the programme. The study demonstrated benefit to the introduction of the mindfulness strategies taught on the course using the quantitative methods and qualitative interviews but this was not supported by the findings relating to cortisol levels (although this is also affected by working shift patterns, which applied to many of the participants).

Where standards of care already exist, the implementation of a new way of working might be evaluated using an audit, although as we saw in the section on evaluation research (Chapter 6, pages 147–150) audit is often constrained in what it can tell us about how and what to improve.

Chapter summary

This chapter provides a sample of the debate about evidence-based nursing practice. We have seen that the adoption of research evidence is complicated by issues such as: identifying a clinical problem; identifying research to address the problem; assessing the quality of the research; considering the quality and applicability of the research as well as the potential for other forms of evidence; and the need to pay due consideration to the needs and preferences of the individuals the evidence will affect.

Evidently this chapter has established that research is only a means to an end and that end is providing the evidence to support improved patient care. In this chapter we have further established that the route to improved care lies not in the blind, uninformed acceptance of the findings of research, but in conscientious and informed appraisal of evidence applied thoughtfully and appreciatively.

Activities: brief outline answers

Activity 7.2   Critical thinking (page 159)

Ideas such as generalisability suggest that some research undertaken in one population might not apply in other populations which are not broadly similar, while notions such as competence and freedom from coercion, and indeed the Mental Capacity Act, highlight that people can if they wish make choices professionals consider not to be good ones.

Activity 7.4   Evidence-based practice and research (page 162)

This activity should show you that some sources of information are not as well informed as others. The pressures on the newspaper journalist are to produce stories and sell papers and not necessarily to inform practice. The motivation for the professional source of information is to inform policy and practice and therefore the paper will be written in professional and considered language. The different emphases for the stories will consequently have a big impact not only on what the authors write but also its accuracy and pertinence to practice.

Further reading

Aveyard, H and Sharp, P (2017) *A Beginner's Guide to Evidence Based Practice in Health and Social Care* (3rd edn). London: Open University Press/McGraw-Hill.

A comprehensive introduction to evidence-based practice with some good links to further sources in the appendix.

Ellis, P (2019) *Evidence-Based Practice in Nursing* (4th edn). London: Sage.

See especially the final chapter on getting evidence into practice.

National Institute for Health and Care Excellence (NICE) (2018) *Practical Steps to Improving the Quality of Care and Services Using NICE Guidance.* London: NICE. Available online at: **https://www.nice.org.uk/Media/Default/About/what-we-do/Into-practice/Practical-steps-improving-quality-of-care-and-services-using-NICE-guidance.pdf** (accessed 5 November 2021).

Standing, M (2020) *Clinical Judgement and Decision Making for Nursing Students* (4th edn). London: Sage.

Guides you through ten aspects of nurses' clinical decision making (e.g. systematic, standardised), which are informed by different types of evidence, including research.

Useful websites

www.evidence.nhs.uk Clinical and non-clinical evidence and best practice website from the NHS.

www.nice.org.uk The website of the National Institute for Health and Care Excellence.

www.sign.ac.uk The Scottish Intercollegiate Guidelines Network (SIGN) develops evidence-based clinical practice guidelines for the NHS in Scotland.

www.casp-uk.net/ The Critical Appraisal Skills Programme website, which contains lots of help and guidance on how to appraise research.

https://jbi.global/ The Joanna Briggs Institute a good source of evidence-based practice information and critiquing tools

Glossary

anthropology: the study of humans and human behaviours.

association: a potential causal connection between two variables.

autonomy: the ability to make choices for oneself.

average: the common name of the arithmetic mean, which is the sum of all the observations in a dataset divided by the number of observations.

behavioural bias: bias that occurs when people within a study behave in a given manner because of some underlying reason that usually affects all similar individuals.

beneficence: the ethical principle of doing good.

bias: in the context of research, anything in the design or undertaking of a study that causes an untruth to occur in the study potentially affecting the outcome of the study. See also *measurement bias; recall bias; response bias; selection bias.*

blinding: the process of hiding from either the participant (single-blind) or both the participant and the researchers (double-blind) which arm of a study (usually a randomised controlled trial) a participant is allocated to. Also known as masking.

bracketing: also referred to as epoching; the process of putting all of your preconceptions about a topic to one side to allow the exploration of a topic as if you were naive about it. This only applies to some forms of phenomenology.

causality: a term used as short-hand for cause and effect.

closed question: a question that requires a limited range of responses such as 'yes' or 'no'.

co-create: work together with all participants in a study to create the outcomes of the study, as in create a new way of working together.

coercion: the application of pressure on someone in order to influence the decision that person makes.

competence: also known as mental competence; the ability to understand and process a decision in a reasonable manner.

confounding: occurs when alternative explanations for an outcome in a study are not accounted for. Confounding variables are always independently associated with both the exposure and the outcome being measured. For example, an increased risk of cancer of the pancreas is associated with both smoking and coffee drinking, and smokers tend to drink more coffee than non-smokers.

consequentialist ethics: the school of ethical thought that states that the consequences of an action (achieving the greater good) are more important than the action itself.

control/control arm: the arm of a randomised controlled trial to which the intervention under research is not applied. People in this arm of a randomised controlled trial are otherwise treated in the same way as people in the intervention arm. This allows the researchers to be sure that the intervention being studied causes the outcome they are measuring.

convenience sample: a sample taken from a set of individuals who are easily accessed.

correlation: an apparent association (relationship) between two variables. A positive correlation occurs in situations when a rise in the independent variable causes an increase in the dependent, while a negative correlation occurs when a rise in the value of the independent variable causes a decrease in the dependent.

credible/credibility: believable. A term used in qualitative research to suggest that the research undertaken actually answers what it set out to answer because of the quality of the way in which the research has been done.

critical appraisal: the structured and thoughtful examination of the quality of something, such as a piece of research to ascertain the level of faith you can place in its findings.

data saturation: the point during data collection for a qualitative study at which no more new ideas or observations are emerging from the people being studied.

deductive: research that sets out to prove an existing idea or hypothesis. The research sets out to explore the truthfulness of the original idea.

deep: see *thick*.

dependability: is a qualitative criterion which means the study is credible.

dependent variable: the outcome variable of the study that occurs as a result of the independent variable having occurred (also called the outcome).

descriptive phenomenology: the study of the essence of being that seeks to apply no interpretation; that is, phenomenology that literally just describes the phenomenon of interest.

descriptive statistics: statistics used to describe the frequencies and patterns of numbers within a dataset.

ecological study: observational studies undertaken at population level of a particular variable and sometimes a change in a dependent variable following a population-level change in independent variable.

emic: taking the insider view – seeing the world from someone else's point of view.

empirical: the notion of discovering new things using the senses or, in the case of research, different methods.

epidemiology: the study of diseases and their treatments from a population perspective.

epistemology: the philosophy of knowledge.

epoching: see *bracketing.*

equivalence studies: comparative studies that compare a new treatment to the current best treatment rather than a placebo.

essence: the nature of something.

ethnography/ethnographic study: the study of the cultures, beliefs and practice of a group.

etic: the outsider's view of something.

experimental: a way of testing a hypothesis through comparison.

exposure: see *independent variable.*

external validity: see *generalisability.*

field notes: where the researcher keeps notes of observations and feelings when collecting data to prompt them when analysing data.

first-person perspective: a view of the world as the individual sees and experiences it.

fixed cohort: the name given to one of the groups in an experimental study recruited according to set criteria which are not changeable later in the study.

gatekeeper: in the research sense, someone from within a group who helps a researcher gain access to the group in order to undertake a study.

generalise/generalisability: the ability of the findings of a study to be extrapolated to the wider population.

grounded theory: a systematic qualitative research methodology which generates a theory of understanding of a phenomenon.

Hawthorne effect: occurs when people respond in the manner in which they believe they should when confronted by a researcher asking questions. The Hawthorne effect can bias a study.

hermeneutics: the interpretation and understanding of language.

homogeneous: the same.

hypothesis: an idea that quantitative research sets out to prove (plural: hypotheses).

incidence: the number of new instances of an event (e.g. an illness) in a given period of time. It sounds like the word 'incident' and, indeed, shares the meaning of a new occurrence.

independent variable: the causal variable in a study, which may be manipulated during a study (also called the exposure).

inductive: the process of developing a theory or hypothesis by first collecting and examining the evidence and seeing where this leads.

inferential statistics: statistics that are used to draw conclusions about the level of association between two or more variables within a study.

interactionist: a philosophical approach that is concerned with how individuals view the world and how they operate in it.

internal consistency: occurs when a respondent answers the same question, perhaps posed in a different way, consistently throughout a survey.

interpretative phenomenological analysis: interpretative phenomenology that takes account of the fact that the interpretation applied is actually an interpretation of the participant's interpretation of his or her own experience.

interpretative phenomenology: phenomenology that attempts to apply an interpretation or understanding to the data collected from the research participants.

inter-rater reliability: the ability of a research tool to show the same rating when used by more than one person (inter – between; rater – person doing using the measure, doing the rating) (see *reliability/reliable*).

interventional: generally applied in quantitative research when an intentional intervention is applied to a research subject in order to measure the effect of the intervention.

iterative: a sort of trial-and-error approach where each attempt at doing something learns from the previous attempt (iteration) so that a clear and useful method for undertaking the task emerges.

justice: to do with acting fairly so that people are treated generally in the same way.

masking: see *blinding.*

mean: also called the average; the sum of all the observations in a dataset divided by the number of observations.

measurement bias: bias that occurs when something is measured incorrectly in a consistent manner.

median: the middle value of an ordered set of observations.

member checking: the process of checking the interpretation of the content of an interview or focus group with the participant(s) to establish the trustworthiness or validity of the understanding the researcher has come to about what s/he has heard.

mental capacity: also referred to as capacity; the ability to retain and understand information needed to make a decision.

meta-analysis: the process of collating the statistics from a number of studies and re-analysing it as one dataset.

methodologies: the broad approaches to research that provide the general framework of the enquiry.

methods: in the sense they are used in this book, the specific tools used to collect data during the research process, e.g. a questionnaire.

mixed methods research: research which uses a variety of methods to collect data in an attempt to increase validity and reliability; see also *triangulation.*

mode: the most frequently occurring number in a dataset.

mortality rate: the death rate in a given population.

non-consequentialist: a view of ethics whereby the action is more important than the outcome. Doing the right thing is therefore seen as more important than what happens as a consequence.

non-experimental: research which does not use comparison to test cause and effect.

non-maleficence: the ethical principle of avoiding doing harm, perhaps better thought of as 'first do no harm'.

null hypothesis: a term whereby a hypothesis is posed as the opposite of what the researchers actually expect to find. Null hypotheses are posed for statistical reasons.

observational studies: studies that involve observation, which in quantitative research is usually quite structured and in qualitative research much less so. Observational studies do not involve an intervention on the part of the researcher.

open question: a question that does not appear to suggest an answer, allowing respondents to give whatever answer they think of.

outcome: see *dependent variable.*

paradigm: in the sense that this term is applied in the book, the philosophical position that is taken within the research.

participant observation: observing the functioning of a group from within the group.

peer review: a common practice in good-quality journals whereby submitted articles are reviewed by subject experts for their accuracy – peer review is usually undertaken without the identity of the writer being disclosed to the reviewers to avoid bias.

period prevalence: the amount of the disease exposure in a given population over a defined period of time.

phenomenology: a research methodology within qualitative research concerned with understanding an experience from the point of view of someone experiencing the phenomenon of interest.

placebo: an inactive form of a treatment used as a comparison in experiments involving new treatments or interventions.

placebo effect: a potentially noticeable improvement in someone's condition that is not due to any active intervention. The improvement is, in fact, the result of what is probably a psychological response to being paid attention.

point prevalence: the amount of whatever is being measured present in the population of interest at this moment in time.

prevalence/prevalent: the amount of a disease/exposure in a defined population at a given point in time.

probability/probabilities: a term used in inferential statistics – a measure of the likelihood of something occurring by chance.

probability sampling: sampling that gives everyone in the study population the same chance of being selected for a study as long as they meet the inclusion criteria. When large enough, such sampling produces results that are generalisable to the population from which the sample is drawn.

prospective: going forward in time.

purposive: a method of sampling within qualitative research whereby people are chosen for inclusion because they meet the purpose of the study. This means they have experience of the phenomenon being studied.

qualitative paradigm: a position associated with the social and psychological sciences. People using this paradigm are interested in discovering truths about how people experience the world and why.

quantitative paradigm: a position that views the world in a more conventionally scientific sense. People using this paradigm are interested in proving associations, correlations and cause and effect.

randomised controlled trial (RCT): a specific form of experiment that is used in the clinical setting in order to compare the usefulness of two or more interventions.

range: the difference between the largest and smallest observations of a dataset.

rapid review: a research methodology which rapidly appraises a service or process, usually using multiple research methods in order to understand the service and design service improvements.

recall bias: bias that occurs when individuals in a study have to rely on their memory in order to answer certain questions. Such biases are created when people who are ill, or have another reason to remember an exposure, are better at recalling events than people who are not ill.

reflexive/reflexivity: the conscious engagement on the part of the researcher in being open to and expressing his or her own biases and opinions that may affect the carrying out and interpretation of the research.

regression to the mean: occurs when people's test scores move from the extremes towards the average when tested a second time.

relevance: in the qualitative sense, this refers to the extent to which the findings of a study might be applied outside the context of the original research.

reliability/reliable: whether a method of data collection, or measurement, will repeatedly give the same results if used by the same person more than once or by two or more people (see *inter-rater reliability*) when measuring the same phenomenon.

representative: the amount of similarity between a study sample and the population from which it is drawn.

research process: a structured approach to asking a research question that is then addressed in a methodical, structured, scientific manner.

response bias: bias that occurs when individuals respond to a question within a study in a particular way because they think that the answer they are giving is what the researcher wants to hear.

retrospective: looking back in time.

rich: see *thick*.

rigour/rigorous: a term used in qualitative research that suggests that the research process has been undertaken in a well-thought-through, well-explained and transparent manner.

sampling bias: bias that occurs when the selection of a sample for a study may exclude certain groups of people in a systematic manner; for example, an online survey will exclude all those people who do not have internet access.

selection bias: bias as a result of an action occurring on one side of a study and not the other. So if researchers were allowed to decide which participants had which intervention in a study, it is possible that they might select patients they thought would do better in the study or try harder to follow a regime – this would be called selection bias.

semi-structured interview: an interview that is partially guided using something like a topic guide or predetermined list of questions.

sensitivity: a measure of the ability of a test to detect a positive result when a result is in truth positive.

sham treatment/intervention: a fake (placebo) treatment used as a comparison for a new treatment in an experiment such as a randomised controlled trial.

structuralist: a philosophical approach concerned with how individuals behave within a group, allowing an understanding of how group cultures are formed and operate.

subjective: a word used to demonstrate that people see the world in different ways, from their own personal perspective.

symbolic interactionism: the study of micro-scale social interactions.

systematic review: a review of the research literature on a given topic which is undertaken using a defined process covering a predetermined number of years of the literature.

tacit knowledge: knowledge that is so deeply embedded that people often forget they have it. It is known to people within a group and does not need explanation within the context of that group, but may be unknown to outsiders.

temporal effect: an effect that makes sense over a period of time, such as a reduction in pain over the few minutes following a kick to the shin.

temporal sequence: the logical order of cause and effect (exposure causing disease and not vice versa).

testing effects: occur when research participants improve their own situation by efforts; this adds to the effect of a research intervention.

theoretical sampling: a method of sampling that occurs as researchers build new theories and ideas from the data they have collected and test these theories by interviewing more subjects to see if the new theories still hold true. Usually only a feature of grounded theory research. Also called 'handy sampling'.

theory: an understanding about an issue that has been derived by collecting evidence.

thick: a term used in qualitative research to denote the fact that the data collected are in-depth, deep, and rich in meaning.

topic guides: short lists of questions to be used as a way of keeping the interviewer focused on the purpose of the interview while also allowing some flexibility.

transferability: the applicability of qualitative research findings to other similar situations.

triangulation: as it applies to research is the use of more than one methodology or method for the collection of research data in an attempt to increase the validity and reliability of a study (see *mixed methods research*).

uncertainty principle: the starting point for all research – because we are uncertain about the answer to a specific question, we undertake research to try to remove the uncertainty.

unstructured interview: an interview that is conducted with few, if any, guiding questions. These interviews are usually very exploratory in nature.

utilitarian ethics: a school of ethical thought that states that the consequences of an action (achieving the greater good) are more important than the action itself.

validity/valid: the ability of a method (or data collection technique) to measure what it is supposed to be measuring. For example, we know that a thermometer (if placed correctly for long enough) will measure temperature, but it is not easy to be certain that a questionnaire designed to measure quality of life does so because of the difficulty of defining what quality of life is.

variable: literally, something that varies, such as eye colour or age. In the sense of research it refers to the thing being explored within the study.

verbatim: word for word, literally 'as something was said'.

References

Abete, I, Zulet, MA, Goyenechea, E, Blazquez, V, de Arce Borda, AM, de Munain, AL and Martinez, A (2018) Association of lifestyle, inflammatory factors, and dietary patterns with the risk of suffering a stroke: a case-control study. *Nutritional Neuroscience*, 12 (1): 70–8.

Adams, WC (2010) Conducting semi-structured interviews, in Wholey, JS, Hatry, HP and Newcomer, K (eds) *Handbook of Practical Program Evaluation* (3rd edn). San Francisco: John Wiley.

Ahlstedt, C, Eriksson Lindvall, C, Holmström, IK, Muntlin Athlin, Å (2019) What makes registered nurses remain in work? An ethnographic study. *International Journal of Nursing Studies*, 89: 32–8.

Althubaiti, A (2016) Information bias in health research: definition, pitfalls, and adjustment methods. *Journal of Multidisciplinary Healthcare*, 9: 211–17.

Ansar, A, Johansson, F, Vásquez, L, Schulze, M and Vaughn, T (2017) Challenges in access to health care among involuntary migrants in Germany: a case study of migrants' experiences in Oldenburg, Lower Saxony. *International Migration*, 55 (2): 97–108.

Bailey, C, Hewison, A, Karasouli, E, Staniszewska, S and Munday, D (2016) Hospital care following emergency admission: a critical incident case study of the experiences of patients with advanced lung cancer and chronic obstructive pulmonary disease. *Journal of Clinical Nursing*, 25 (15): 2168–79.

Beauchamp, T and Childress, J (2013) *Principles of Biomedical Ethics* (7th edn). Oxford: Oxford University Press.

Berk, M, Otmar, R, Dean, O et al. (2015) The use of mixed methods in drug discovery: integrating qualitative methods into clinical trials, in Tohen, M, Bowden, AC, Nierenberg, AA et al. (eds) *Clinical Trial Design Challenges in Mood Disorders*. New York: Elsevier.

Bhavsar, V, Fusar-Poli, P and McGuire, P (2017) Neighbourhood deprivation is positively associated with detection of the ultra-high risk (UHR) state for psychosis in South East London. *Schizophrenia Research*. http://dx.doi.org/10.1016/j.schres.2017.06.006

Biros, M (2018) Capacity, vulnerability, and informed consent for research. *The Journal of Law, Medicine & Ethics*, 46 (1): 72–8.

Blackhouse, T, Killett, A, Penhale, B and Gray R (2016) The use of non-pharmacological interventions for dementia behaviours in care homes: findings from four in-depth, ethnographic case studies. *Age and Ageing*, 45 (6): 856–63.

Booth, A (2009) Using evidence in practice: research or evaluation? Does it matter? *Health Information and Libraries Journal*, 26: 255–58.

Bowling, A (2014) *Research Methods in Health: Investigating Health and Health Services* (4th edn). Maidenhead: Open University Press.

Bradbury-Jones, C, Sambrook, S and Irvine, F (2009) The phenomenological focus group: an oxymoron? *Journal of Advanced Nursing*, 65 (3): 663–71.

Bradshaw, A and Price, L (2007) Rectal suppository insertion: the reliability of the evidence as a basis for nursing. *Practice Journal of Clinical Nursing*, 16: 98–103.

Brew, B, Shannon, C, Storey, L, Boyd, A and Mulholland, C (2017) A qualitative phenomenological analysis of the subjective experience and understanding of the at risk mental state. *International Journal of Qualitative Studies on Health and Well-Being*, 12 (1): 1342504.

Brinkmann, S and Kvale, S (2014) *InterViews: Learning the Craft of Qualitative Research Interviewing* (3rd edn). London: Sage.

Broberg, G, Wang, J, Östberg, AL, Adolfson, A, Nemes, S, Sparen, P and Strander, B (2018) Socio-economic and demographic determinants affecting participation in the Swedish cervical screening program: a population-based case-control study. *Public Library of Science One.* https://doi.org/10.1371/journal.pone.0190171

Burgoon, JD, Guerrero, LK and Floyd, K (2016) *Non-Verbal Communication.* Oxford: Routledge.

Callwood, A, Cooke, D, Bolger, S, Lemanska, A and Allen, H (2018) The reliability and validity of multiple mini interviews (MMIs) in values based recruitment to nursing, midwifery and paramedic practice programmes: findings from an evaluation study. *International Journal of Nursing Studies*, 77: 138–44.

Campbell, DT and Fiske, DW (1959) Convergent and discriminant validation by the multitrait-multimethod matrix. *Psychological Bulletin*, 56 (2): 81–105.

Care Quality Commission (2015) Delivering cost effective care in the NHS: working together to develop how CQC will assess the use of resources in NHS acute trusts. Available online at: www.cqc.org.uk/sites/default/files/20151028_delivering_cost_effective_care_in_the_NHS.pdf (accessed 13 July 2021).

Carey, MA and Asbury, J-O (2016) *Focus Group Research.* London: Routledge.

Carr, W and Kemmis, S (1986) *Becoming Critical: Education, Knowledge and Action Research.* Lewes: Falmer.

Celentano, M and Szklo, DD (2019) *Gordis Epidemiology.* Philadelphia: Elsevier.

Chen, HM, Chen, VCH, Wang, TN, Lu, ML, Huang, YC, Dewey, M, Lee, JKW and Tsai, CP (2018) Diseases of the pancreas and suicide mortality: a nationwide nested case-control study among patients with mental health disorders in Taiwan. *General Hospital Psychiatry*, 50: 45–50.

Chyung, SY, Roberts, K, Swanson, I and Hankinson, A (2017) Evidence-based survey design: the use of a midpoint on the Likert scale. *Performance Improvement*, 56 (10): 15–23.

Clwyd, A and Hart, T (2013) A review of the NHS hospitals: putting patients back in the picture. Available online at: www.gov.uk/government/publications/nhs-hospitals-complaints-system-review (accessed 8 August 2015).

Coffey, A (2018) *Doing Ethnography* (2nd edn). London: Sage.

Creswell, JW and Creswell, JD (2018) *Research Design: Qualitative, Quantitative, and Mixed Methods Approaches* (5th edn). London: Sage.

Creswell, J and Poth, CN (2017) *Qualitative Inquiry and Research Design: Choosing among Five Approaches* (4th edn). Thousand Oaks: Sage.

Crotty, M (1998) *The Foundations of Social Research: Meaning and Perspective in the Research Process.* London: Sage.

Cypress, BS (2017) Rigor or reliability and validity in qualitative research: perspectives, strategies, reconceptualization, and recommendations. *Dimensions of Critical Care Nursing,* 36 (4): 253–63.

Delamont, S and Atkinson, P (2018) The ethics of ethnography, in Iphofen, R and Tolich, M (eds) *The Sage Handbook of Qualitative Research Ethics.* London: Sage.

Desborough, J, Banfield, M, Phillips, C and Mills, J (2016) The process of patient enablement in general practice nurse consultations: a grounded theory study. *Journal of Advanced Nursing,* 73 (5): 1085–96.

Dowrick, AS, Wootten, AC, Murphy, DG and Costello, AJ (2015) 'We used a validated questionnaire': What does this mean and is it an accurate statement in urologic research? *Urology,* 85 (6): 1304–10.

Doyle, L, McCabe, C, Keogh, B, Brady, A and McCann, M (2020) An overview of the qualitative descriptive design within nursing research. *Journal of Research in Nursing.* 25 (5): 443–55.

Duko, B, Geja, E, Oltaye, Z, Belayneh, F, Kedir, A and Gebire, M (2019) Triage knowledge and skills among nurses in emergency units of Specialized Hospital in Hawassa, Ethiopia: cross sectional study. *BMC Research Notes,* 12: 21.

Ekirapa-Kiracho, E, Kananura, RM, Tetui, M, Namazzi, G, Mutebi, A, George, A et al. (2017) Effect of a participatory multisectoral maternal and newborn intervention on maternal health service utilization and newborn care practices: a quasi-experimental study in three rural Ugandan districts. *Global Health Action,* 10 (S4): 18–28.

Ellis, P (2018) The language of research (part 18): research methodologies: rapid appraisals (2). *Wounds UK,* 14 (4): 108–9.

Ellis, P (2019) *Evidence-Based Practice in Nursing* (4th edn). London: Sage.

Ellis, PA and Cairns, HS (2001) Renal impairment in elderly patients with hypertension and diabetes. *Quarterly Journal of Medicine,* 94: 261–5.

Elo, S, Kääriäinen, M, Kanste, O, Pölkki, T, Utriainen, K and Kyngäs, H (2014) *Qualitative Content Analysis: A Focus on Trustworthiness.* London: Sage Open. Available online at: http://sgo.sagepub.com/content/4/1/2158244014522633.full-text.pdf+html (accessed 8 August 2015). doi:10.1177/2158244014522633

Englund, H (2020) Using unfolding case studies to develop critical thinking skills in baccalaureate nursing students: A pilot study. *Nurse Education Today,* 93: 104542.

Engward, H and Davis, G (2015) Being reflexive in qualitative grounded theory: discussion and application of a model of reflexivity. *Journal of Advanced Nursing,* 71 (7): 1530–8.

Eslami Akbar, R, Elahi, N, Mohammadi, E and Fallahi Khoshknab, M (2017) How do the nurses cope with job stress? a study with grounded theory approach. *Journal of Caring Sciences*, 6 (3): 199–211.

Farrell, C, Walshe, C and Molassiotis, A (2017) Are nurse-led chemotherapy clinics really nurse-led? An ethnographic study. *International Journal of Nursing Studies*, 69: 1–8.

Fink, A (2019) *Conducting Research Literature Reviews* (5th edn). London: Sage.

Glaser, B and Strauss, A (1967) *The Discovery of Grounded Theory*. Chicago, IL: Aldine.

Griffith, JW, Messersmith, EE, Gillespie BW, Wiseman, JB, Flynn, KE, Kirkali, Z et al. (2018) Reasons for seeking clinical care for lower urinary tract symptoms: a mixed methods study. *Journal of Urology*, 199 (2): 528–35.

Grove, SK and Cipher, D (2020) *Statistics for Nursing Research* (3rd edn). London: Elsevier.

Groves, E, Rayner, K and Muncer, S (2017) 'It's good, they're like me; the same but different'. An interpretative phenomenological analysis of the identities of women with Down's syndrome. *Journal of Applied Research in Intellectual Disabilities*. doi:10.1111/jar.12425

Hales, P, White, A, Eden, A, Hurst, R, Moore, S, Riotto, C and Achour, N (2020) A case study of a collaborative allied health and nursing crisis response, *Journal of Interprofessional Care*, 34 (5): 614-21.

Hancock, DR and Algozzine, B (2017) *Doing Case Study Research: A Practical Guide for Beginning Researchers*. New York: Teachers College Press.

Health Research Authority (HRA) (2014) Consent and participant information guidance. Available online at: www.hra-decisiontools.org.uk/consent (accessed 10 October 2021).

Heath Hearn, J, Finlay, KA, Fine, PA and Cotter, I (2017) Neuropathic pain in a rehabilitation setting after spinal cord injury: an interpretative phenomenological analysis of inpatients' experiences. *Nature; Spinal Cord Series and Cases*, 3 (17083). doi: 10.1038/s41394-017-0032-9.

Henwood, KL and Pidgeon, NR (1992) Qualitative research and psychological theorising. *British Journal of Psychology*, 83 (1): 97–112.

Hoe, NY and Nambiar, R (1985) Is preoperative shaving really necessary? *Annals of Academic Medicine Singapore*, 14: 700–4.

Howlett M (2021) Looking at the 'field' through a Zoom lens: methodological reflections on conducting online research during a global pandemic. *Qualitative Research*. doi:10.1177/1468794120985691

Hyett, N, Kenny, A and Dickson-Swift, V (2014) Methodology or method? A critical review of qualitative case study reports. *International Journal of Qualitative Studies on Health and Well-Being*, 9 (10). doi:10.3402/qhw.v9.23606

Jangland, E, Kitson, A and Muntlin Athlin, Å (2016) Patients with acute abdominal pain describe their experiences of fundamental care across the acute care episode: a multi-stage qualitative case study. *Journal of Advanced Nursing*, 72 (4): 791–801.

Jensen, EJ, Wieling, E and Mendenhall, T (2020) A phenomenological study of clinicians' perspectives on barriers to rural mental health care. *Journal of Rural Mental Health*, 44 (1): 51–61.

Kaptchuk, TJ and Miller, FG (2015) Placebo effects in medicine. *New England Journal of Medicine*, 373 (1): 8–9.

Kara, H (2018) *Research Ethics in the Real World: Euro-Western and Indigenous Perspectives*. Bristol: Policy Press.

Kemp, JH, Bannon, EM, Mwanja, MM and Tebuseeke, D (2018) Developing a national standard for midwifery mentorship in Uganda. *International Journal of Health Governance*. doi.org/10.1108/IJHG-09-2017-0051

Kvarnstrom, S, Jangland, E and Abrandt Dahlgren, M (2017) Introducing the nurse practitioner into the surgical ward: an ethnographic study of interprofessional teamwork practice. *Scandanavian Journal of Caring Sciences*. doi:10.1111/scs.12507

Lewin, K (1946) Action research and minority problems, in Lewin, GW (ed.) *Researching Social Conflicts: Selected Papers on Group Dynamics*. New York: Harpers.

Leyva-Moral, JM and Feijoo-Cid, M (2017) Participants' safety versus confidentiality: a case study of HIV research. *Nursing Ethics*, 24 (3): 376–80.

Lorhan, S, van der Westhuizen, M and Gossman, S (2015) The role of volunteers at an outpatient cancer center: how do volunteers enhance the patient experience? *Supportive Care in Cancer*, 23 (6): 1597–605.

Lynn, P (2021) *Advances in Longitudinal Survey Methodology*. Hoboken: Wiley.

Matta, C (2019) Qualitative research methods and evidential reasoning. *Philosophy of the Social Sciences*, 49 (5): 385–412.

McLaughlin, H (2008) *Service-User Research in Health and Social Care*. London: Sage.

Moran, D (2000) *Introduction to Phenomenology*. London: Routledge.

Moule, P (2021) *Making Sense of Research in Nursing, Health and Social Care* (7th edn). London: Sage.

Murray, EJ (2021) Editorial: Demystifying the placebo effect. *American Journal of Epidemiology*, 190 (1): 2–9.

National Institute for Health and Care Excellence (2015) Research recommendations: Process and methods guide. Available online at: www.nice.org.uk/Media/Default/About/what-we-do/Science-policy-and-research/research-recommendation-process-methods-guide-2015.pdf (accessed 13 July 2021).

National Institute for Health and Care Excellence (2018) *NICE impact: Cancer*. Available online at: https://www.nice.org.uk/Media/Default/About/what-we-do/Into-practice/measuring-uptake/nice-impact-cancer.pdf (accessed 13 January 2022).

National Institute for Health Research (2013) *Good Practice Guidance for Involving People with Experience of Mental Health Problems in Research*. London: NIHR.

Nicholson, WJ, Perkel, G and Selikoff, IJ (1982) Occupational exposure to asbestos: population at risk and projected mortality, 1980–2030. *American Journal of Industrial Medicine*, 982 (3): 259.

NMC (Nursing and Midwifery Council) (2018a) *Future Nurse: Standards of Proficiency for Registered Nurses*. London: NMC.

NMC (Nursing and Midwifery Council) (2018b) *The Code: Professional Standards of Practice and Behaviour for Nurses, Midwives and Nursing Associates.* London: NMC.

O'Leary, Z (2021) *The Essential Guide to Doing Your Research Project* (3rd edn). London: Sage.

Orellana-Rios, CL, Radbruch, L, Kern, M, Regel, YU, Anton, A, Sinclair, S and Schmidt, S (2017) Mindfulness and compassion-oriented practices at work reduce distress and enhance self-care of palliative care teams: a mixed-method evaluation of an 'on the job' program. *BMC Palliative Care*, 17 (3). https://doi.org/10.1186/s12904-017-0219-7

Øvretveit, J (2017) Perspectives: answering questions about quality improvement: suggestions for investigators. *International Journal for Quality in Health Care*, 29 (1): 137–142. https://doi.org/10.1093/intqhc/mzw136

Palladino, R, Vamos, E, Chang, KCM and Millet, C (2017) Impact of a national diabetes risk assessment and screening programme in England: a quasi-experimental study. *The Lancet*, 390 (S3): S65. https://doi.org/10.1016/S0140-6736(17)33000-3

Paltved, C, Morcke, AM and Nusaeus, P (2015) Insider action research and the microsystem of a Danish surgical ward. *Action Research* 1476750315592937, first published on 1 July 2015. doi:10.1177/14767 50315592937

Pan, R, Zhou, M, Cai, H, Guo, Y, Zhan, L, Mei, L et al. (2018) A randomized controlled trial of a modified wheelchair arm-support to reduce shoulder pain in stroke patients. *Clinical Rehabilitation*, 32 (1): 37–47.

Parahoo, K (2014) *Nursing Research: Principles, Process and Issues* (3rd edn). London: Palgrave Macmillan.

Patrick, J (1973) *A Glasgow Gang Observed.* London: Methuen.

Patton, M (1986) *How to Use Qualitative Methods in Evaluation.* London: Sage.

Pederson, B, Delmar, C, Falkmer, U and Grønkjær, M (2016) Bridging the gap between interviewer and interviewee: developing an interview guide for individual interviews by means of a focus group. *Scandanavian Journal of Caring Sciences*, 30 (3): 631–8.

Peterson, ER and Barron, KA (2007) How to get focus groups talking: new ideas that will stick. *International Journal of Qualitative Methods*, 6 (3): 140–4.

Petrie, A and Sabin, C (2020) *Medical Statistics at a Glance* (4th edn). London: Wiley-Blackwell.

Polit DF and Beck, CT (2020) *Nursing Research: Generating and Assessing Evidence for Nursing Practice* (11th edn). London: Wolters Kluwer/Lippincott Williams & Wilkins.

Popay, J, Rogers, A and Williams, G (1998) Rationale and standards for the systematic review of qualitative literature in health services research. *Qualitative Health Research*, 8 (3): 341–51.

Pope, C and Mays, N (2020) *Foundations of Nursing Research* (4th edn). London: Wiley-Blackwell.

Powney, J and Watts, M (1987) *Interviewing in Educational Research.* London: Routledge & Kegan Paul.

Ramezani, M, Ahmadi, F, Mohammadi, E and Kazemnejad, A (2017) The grounded theory of trust building. *Nursing Ethics.* https://doi.org/10.1177/0969733017734411

Reay, G, Raffin Bouchal, S and Rankin, JA (2016) Staying theoretically sensitive when conducting grounded theory research. *Nurse Researcher,* 24 (1): 26–30.

Rivaz, M, Shokrollahi, P and Ebadi, A (2019) Online focus group discussions: an attractive approach to data collection for qualitative health research. *Journal of Nursing Practice Today,* 6 (1): 1-3.

Roulstin, K (2014) Analysing interviews, in Flick, U (ed.) *The Sage Handbook of Qualitative Data Analysis.* London: Sage.

Saad, K, Abdel-Rahman, AA, Elserogy, YM, Al-Atram, AA, El-Houfey, AA, Othman, HAK et al. (2018) Randomized controlled trial of vitamin D supplementation in children with autism spectrum disorder. *Journal of Child Psychology and Psychiatry,* 59 (1): 20–9.

Sackett, DL, Rosenberg, WM, Gray, JA, Haynes, RB and Richardson, WS (1996) Evidence based medicine: what it is and what it isn't. *British Medical Journal,* 312 (7023): 71–2.

Saga, S, Guttormsen, V, Mørkved, S, Norton, C and Seim, A (2015) What characteristics predispose to continence in nursing home residents? A population-based cross-sectional study. *Neurourology and Urodynamics,* 34: 362–7.

Sarantakos, S (2012) *Social Research* (4th edn). London: Palgrave Macmillan.

Sauer, M and Abbotts, C (2018) A new pen device for injection of recombinant human growth hormone: a convenience, functionality and usability evaluation study. *Patient Preference and Adherence,* 12: 27–34.

Sinclair, S, Beamer, K, Hack, TF, McClement, S, Raffin Bouchal, S, Chochinov, HM and Hagen, NA (2016) Sympathy, empathy, and compassion: a grounded theory study of palliative care patients' understandings, experiences, and preferences. *Palliative Medicine,* 31 (5): 437–47.

Smith, J (2016) *Experiencing Phenomenology: An Introduction.* London: Routledge

Smith, SR, Murray, D, Pockney, PG, Bendinelli, C, Draganic, BD and Carroll, R (2018) Tranexamic acid for lower GI hemorrhage: a randomized placebo-controlled clinical trial. *Diseases of the Colon and Rectum,* 61 (1): 99–106.

Spagrud, LJ, Piira, T and von Baeyer, CL (2003) Children's self-report of pain intensity: the Faces Pain Scale – Revised. *American Journal of Nursing,* 103 (12): 62–4.

Stone Sunstein, B and Chiseri-Strater, E (2012) *Field Working: Reading and Writing Research* (4th edn). Boston: Bedford/St Martins.

Strauss, A and Corbin, J (1990) *Basics of Qualitative Research.* Thousand Oaks: Sage.

Streubert, HJ and Carpenter, DR (2010) *Qualitative Research in Nursing: Advancing the Humanistic Imperative* (5th edn). London: Lippincott Williams & Wilkins.

Taub, S, Krivoy, A, Whiskey, E and Shergill, SS (2021) New approaches to antipsychotic medication adherence – safety, tolerability and acceptability, *Expert Opinion on Drug Safety.* https://doi.org/10.1080/14740338.2021.1983540

Tod, A (2015) Interviewing, in Gerrish, K and Lathlean, J (eds) *The Research Process in Nursing* (7th edn). Oxford: Wiley-Blackwell.

Topping, A (2015) The quantitative–qualitative continuum, in Gerrish, K and Lathlean, J (eds) *The Research Process in Nursing* (7th edn). Oxford: Wiley-Blackwell.

Tørring, B, Gittell, JH, Laursen, M, Rasmussen, BS and Sørensen, EE (2019) Communication and relationship dynamics in surgical teams in the operating room: an ethnographic study. *BMC Health Service Research*, 19 (528). https://doi.org/10.1186/s12913-019-4362-0

USAID (2010) Performance monitoring and evaluation using rapid evaluation methods. Available online at: www.dmeforpeace.org/wp-content/uploads/2017/06/USAID_TIPS- Using20RapidAppraisal20Methods.pdf (accessed 23 January 2018).

Vindrola-Padros, C, Andrews, L, Dowrick, A, Djellouli, N, Fillmore, H, Gonzalez, EB et al. (2020) Perceptions and experiences of healthcare workers during the COVID-19 pandemic in the UK. *BMJ Open*, 10: e040503. doi: 10.1136/bmjopen-2020-040503

Walters, SJ, Campbell, MJ and Machin, D (2021) *Medical Statistics: A Textbook for the Health Sciences* (5th edn). Chichester: John Wiley.

World Medical Association (WMA) (2013) Declaration of Helsinki: ethical principles for medical research involving human subjects. *Journal of the American Medical Association*, 310 (20): 2191–4.

Writing Group for the Women's Health Initiative Investigators (2002) Risks and benefits of estrogen plus progestin in healthy postmenopausal women: principal results from the Women's Health Initiative randomized controlled trial. *Journal of the American Medical Association*, 288 (3): 321–33.

Yakusheva, O and Fletcher, J (2015) Learning from teen childbearing experiences of close friends: evidence using miscarriages as a natural experiment. *Review of Economics and Statistics*, 97 (1): 29–43.

Yin, RK (2018) *Case Study Research and Applications: Design and Methods* (6th edn). Thousand Oaks: Sage.

Zahavi, D (2018) *Phenomenology: The Basics*. London: Routledge.

Index

Note: References in **bold r**efer to the Glossary, *f* refers to figures, *t* to tables.

Hoe, N.Y. 84
homogeneous samples 44, **172**
hormone replacement therapy (HRT) 86
Husserl, E. 39
hypotheses 14, 15–16, 43, 86–87, 87*f*, 93, **172**

incidence 97, **172**
incident cases 103
independent variable 82, 83–86, **172**
inductive reasoning 36–37
inductive research 15–16, 16*f*, 36, **172**
inferential statistics 126, 129–131, 133*f*, **172**
inter-rater reliability 120, **173**
interactionist view 144, **172**
internal consistency 124, **173**
interpretative phenomenological analysis 40, **173**
interpretative phenomenology 39, **173**
interventional research 82, **173**
interviews 57–59
    advantages 62–63
    disadvantages 63–64
    key features 59–62
    video recording 62
interviews, types of 64
    focus group interviews 67
    semi-structured interviews 41–42, 64–65, **176**
    structured interviews 121–122
    unstructured interviews 41–42, 65, **177**
iterative process 33, **173**

Jangland, E. et al. 50
Jensen, E.J. et al. 41
Joanna Briggs Institute (JBB) 163
justice 21, **173**

Kemmis, S. 151
Kemp, J.H. et al. 151

Lancet, The 84
learning features 2–3
Lewin, K. 151, 152*f*
Likert items 117
literature reviews 9, 17–18
logical generalisations 38
Lorhan, S. et al. 143

McLaughlin, H. 22
masking *see* blinding
Matta, C. 140
Mays, N. 38, 46, 62
mean 127, 127*f*, **173**
measurement bias 142, **173**
measures of central tendency 126, 132*t*
    arithmetic mean 127, 127*f*, **170**
    median 127, 127*f*, **173**
    mode 128, 128*f*, **173**
    range 128, **175**
    standard deviation 128–129, 129*f*
median 127, 127*f*, **173**
member checking 67, **173**
mental capacity 23, **173**
meta-analyses 18, **173**

methodological separatism 140
methodologies 5, 33, **173**
    see also qualitative methodologies; quantitative
        methodologies; research methodologies
methods 5, **173**
mixed methods research 2, 141, **173**
mode 128, 128*f*, **173**
mortality rate 103, **173**
Moule, P. 160
multiple methods 139–140

Nambiar, R. 84
natural experiments *see* quasi-experiments
needs assessment 147–148
NICE (National Institute for Health and Care
    Excellence) 9, 10, 34
NMC (Nursing and Midwifery Council) 23
    Standards of Proficiency for Registered Nurses 2,
        33–34, 73–74, 111, 160
non-consequentialist approach 21, **173**
non-experimental studies 82, **174**
non-maleficence 21, **174**
null hypothesis 93, **174**
Nurses' Health Studies 98–99, 99*t*, 100, 101

observation 69
    advantages 72–73
    disadvantages 73
    participant observation 46, 48, 70–73, 72*f*, **174**
observational studies 82, 85, 141, **174**
O'Leary, Z. 74–75
open questions 49, 115, 115*t*, **174**
Orellana-Rios, C.L. et al. 168
outcome *see* dependent variable
outcome evaluation 149
Øvretveit, J. 165

Palladino, R. et al. 89
Paltved, C. et al. 152
paradigms 14, **174**
Parahoo, K. 60–61, 74
parametric/non-parametric data 132–133
    chi-square test 134
    distribution curve 132, 133*f*
    t-test 133–134
participant observation 46, 48, **174**
    advantages 72–73
    dimensions of 72*t*
    disadvantages 73
    key features 70–72
peer review **174**
peer reviewed information 162
period prevalence 104, 105, **174**
personal development plans/portfolios (PDP) 3
Peterson, E.R. 68
phenomenology 13, 17, 38, **174**
    data collection methods 41–42, 58
    data presentation/interpretation 75
    descriptive phenomenology 39
    interpretative phenomenology 39, **173**
    key features 39–40
    sampling 40–41